How Not to Wear Black

and Discover Your True Colors

How Not to Wear Black

and Discover Your True Colors

Jules Standish

BOOKS

Winchester, UK
Washington, USA

First published by O-Books, 2011
O-Books is an imprint of John Hunt Publishing Ltd., Laurel House, Station Approach,
Alresford, Hants, SO24 9JH, UK
office1@o-books.net
www.o-books.com

For distributor details and how to order please visit the 'Ordering' section on our website.

Text copyright: Jules Standish 2010

Copyright permission received from Colourflair to use Personality Questionnaire and responses
and all eye illustrations.

Copyright image of front cover lady belongs to artist Vincent Poole.

ISBN: 978 1 84694 561 8

A CIP catalogue record for this book is available from the British Library.

Design: Stuart Davies

Printed in the UK by CPI Antony Rowe
Printed in the USA by Offset Paperback Mfrs, Inc

We operate a distinctive and ethical publishing philosophy in all
areas of our business, from our global network of authors to
production and worldwide distribution.

CONTENTS

ACKNOWLEDGEMENTS

Thank you O-Books for giving me the opportunity to publish a book that hopes to inspire women and men on colour and how to wear black well.

There are many people who contributed to this book, and my thanks go to Janey Lee Grace for writing such a great foreword, and Diana Moran and Davina Mackail for finding the time to write about their experiences with colour and agreeing to share it.

Thank you to all the wonderful experts in their fields who were happy to help me in my quest to write about black and colour; Alison Standish, Alla Svirinskaya, Theresa Sundt, Victoria Galbraith, Harry Oldfield, Philippa Merivale and Gisele Mir.

To all my clients over the years who have benefited from discovering their true colours and allowing me to gain the insight that has enabled me to write this book. Thank you to those who have allowed me to include personal experiences too, particularly Mel.

Pat Scott Vincent, founder of Colourflair, has been my great teacher and true inspiration for getting the word "out there" about the importance of colour in our lives. Her support, encouragement and love combined with her professional input enabled this book to be written along with Ray.

My thanks to Sarah Jane Burrowes for her in-depth and incredibly detailed eye illustrations that are of vital importance in the self help chapter of the book. Also to the hugely talented artist Vince Poole for his front cover girl image.

Thank you to all my adorable friends for support, encouragement and contributions, in particular Sue, Rachel, Georgie, Trish, Mich, Fee, Charlotte, Karen, Lizzie, Jo, Leslie and Fiona. With my special thanks to Lou and Iain, Fabba Susie and Pip.

Jonathan and Alex provided me with all the computer back up and knowledge to help produce images and pictures for the book and on my website and for creating the website in the first place. Boys, you have done a great job.

…and finally to my children, Becca and Alex for allowing me to write this book during the summer holidays and my darling husband Miles who gave up a whole weekend to sit and read through all the text before being allowed out! Thanks to my lovely mum who has given me the confidence in life to believe I can do anything.

FOREWORD

by radio presenter and author Janey Lee Grace

Oh lucky you! The inspirational Jules Standish has revealed all in this great new book. She knows her stuff this girl and trust me this is your in-road to personal styling and color analysis.

I remember years ago having a consultation with someone who offered a 'color session', she draped a few scarves around my neck, and sent me off with a swatch of insipid colors that I mostly hated. I descended straight back into my safe black.

My experience with Jules was entirely different, it's much more than simply checking what 'season' you are, Jules has done some serious studying on color – based on Johannes Ittens color wheel, She explains how the right colors can stimulate, enhance, inspire or calm us – in short it can be transformational. Being aware and intuitive about color can not only enhance your style, but encourage you to really get in touch with your personality, and harmonize your energy fields. Jules also made me realize that far from being the 'slimming aid' we think wearing black can often make us look fatter!

Without doubt color has a psychological effect on our brain. We all know how our spirits are lifted on a bright sunny day, given that in the UK we aren't usually blessed with the quality of light that the Mediterranean and other countries enjoy for much of the year, if we then wear grays and blacks it can add to our gloom and depression. If we inject some color into our clothing and accessories we can go some way to bringing back the sunshine!

Jules' recommendations are not limited to fashion, she is very conscious of the importance of color in the home too and wrote a fantastic guide to the use of decorative color and interior design for my book' Imperfectly Natural Home'.

I also love the fact that Jules takes the holistic approach. She has one eye on sustainability and is conscious of eco fashion and fabrics, she was quite impressed with my 'charity shop chic' wardrobe and although a few of my impulse vintage bargains didn't flatter me color-wise and had to be recycled back to the charity shop, mostly she was happy to help me mix and match colors and styles. I also love that Jules is passionate about natural skincare and cosmetics too (she's a cracking make-up artist!).

So enjoy this book and may we welcome you especially if you're a 'shades of black and grey only' gal into the wonderful world of color – it really is the new black.

CHAPTER ONE

INTRODUCING YOUR TRUE COLOURS

Are you being true to yourself, wearing the colors you were born to be seen in? Have you unknowingly moved away from your inherited true characteristics? Do you know what they were in the first place?

How would you like to give yourself a transformational color analysis? A once in a lifetime experience, and one of the best investments you will ever make. You will have the chance to find out for yourself not only what colors will make you look healthy and fabulous, but whether black can be worn into old age without you looking and feeling older than your clothes!

Throughout your life, from birth to old age, you will be surrounded by many colors to choose from, but how do you really know which enhance your personality and are in harmony with your individual coloring? What shades will give you the therapeutic benefits physically and emotionally, that will make you look and feel younger and healthier.

What does black do energetically to the physical body? Everyone has an "aura" or energy field and color has powerful affects on emotional needs at different times in ones life. The right colors can make you radiate with health and well being.

You are born with an inherited, genetic, blue print of personality traits and coloring. However, through personal circumstances, challenging situations and emotional difficulties, you may find that you have changed along the way. A naturally extrovert, fun loving person may have had to cope with bereavement or divorce and found themselves reverting to black or dark colors that hide their true nature.

Putting oneself in black when not in this "state" can be very draining. Women often resort to black through illness or trauma, low self esteem and due to being overweight. What they don't realize is that staying in black can hinder their recovery and keep them in their grief or hiding from their fears. Why do people automatically go into black when mourning or depressed? Throughout the ages black has been associated with death and grief, and has had that mystical, dark and sinister edge to it.

In modern times fashion has made it sexy and stylish. It is a wardrobe staple for modern women and men particularly within the business sector. A color to hide behind, feel protected and safe in and sometimes not to be noticed in.

Theresa Sundt the color therapist and artist says "in painting, black is lack of color, which is why it works well for framing as it puts a boundary round pictures, outlining color within them". Black also provides a boundary around people when they do not want to show their colors to the world, or give out any messages. We all need time out and for some people black becomes a valuable shield against society.

Your genetics are the most influential thing when finding the correct colors to suit you. Your eyes hold the key to the color of your skin tone. Do you have the dark crypts and spokes of a true melancholic with cool skin? Can you wear the strong, dynamic make up that only truly suits this coloring?

A true cool melancholic lady will look lovely wearing black, however, there are only a minority of women in the Western world who genuinely have the skin tone and personality to look fabulous in it at any age.

Is it you? Find out by following the self-help guidelines in this book.

Did you also know that by asking some simple personality questions, you can find out what your temperament is. Are you a "sunny sanguine", "patient phlegmatic", a "dynamic choleric" or the "introverted melancholic" that can wear black and not feel tired and washed out by it? Perhaps you show tendencies of more than one personality type. The colors you are wearing should complement your personality, but what happens when you are wearing the wrong colors for your temperament?

Many great psychologists including Jung and Steiner have written about temperaments and their impact on our personalities. It was Hippocrates who first established the 4 different "humors" (temperaments) and how they affect our skin tones.

As a color black is highly controversial and emotive - it gives the illusion of making women look slimmer. Designers who adorn themselves in black season after season brainwash us through the media, that black is always "the" color to be seen in. From a styling point of view, it is not just about getting your body dressed in the right shapes. It is also about making sure your face is not being aged dramatically or being made to look unhealthy by wearing the wrong colors.

Celebrity fashion is followed by the masses, and many high profile personalities wear black and influence our culture, which is obsessed with youth. From a beauty perspective over a certain age, the skin starts to lose its color, lines and wrinkles start to appear, with shadows under the chin and dark circles around the eyes being highlighted, and to crown it all roots in the hair! Black will enhance all these negatives on the wrong skin tone. How would you feel if you thought black was ageing your face by ten years?

Women now more than any other generation are looking at ways to keep from ageing and look younger. Color has such a transformational effect and does a natural face-lift instantly when correct shades are put up to the face. Why spend lots of money on cosmetic surgery when getting the colors right can do the same job for relatively little?

Also, it's not just women. Men have become more fashion conscious and spend money and time on their looks too. Black can be very damaging for men, as they are not able to counteract the negative effects with make-up.

What does black do for you? Does it truly suit your nature and coloring? If it is detrimental to you then I will show you how to continue to wear it in flattering ways that are not ageing to your face, or draining to you energetically.

Discovering your true colors can be powerful as they have the ability to affect you on many levels. Why do some people really shine wearing bright colors and others look simply overpowered by them? Ever had one of those days where people tell you how well you look? That's probably because you are wearing one of your true colors.

This book will help to guide you through understanding your individual temperament and show you which harmonious colors suit you. Your true colors will be revealed, and enable you to live the rest of your life knowing that you are supporting your personality, and making the most of your image and looks.

About The Color System

There is a great deal of contradictory material written about color analysis. Although hair and eye color are an important part of the overall impression created by coloring, they are not the deciding factor when you are finding the colors that flatter and bring a healthy glow to your complexion. Categorizing people in this way is called "Type Analysis" a system based upon the general appearance according to stereotypes. However, unless you fall into the "classic" type of a seasons coloring this system is not beneficial as hair in particular, is an extremely unreliable guide to the underlying skin tone.

The aim of color analysis is to provide accurate results. This means taking into account your personality, health, and coloring. Understanding your genetics is vital. It will provide you with the key to your harmonizing colors; the ones that will bring out the best of your features through the clothes that you wear and the make up that you use.

We all inherit our coloring from a close relation, normally either our parents or our grandparents. Eye color, skin tone, hair and personality temperament are all made up of inherited genes. It may be that you have a combination of coloring from different family members and this is what makes you an individual.

The color analysis system described in this book, was devised over 20 years ago, by Pat Scott Vincent, the founder of Colourflair. Her work was based on Bernice Kentner's methods, originating over 30 years ago in America. Pat is an inspirational teacher and one of the original members of the International Federation of Image Consultants, and past president.

The Colourflair system is different to "Type Analysis"; it is holistic, and based on a series of tests to determine skin tone: looking at your personality, eye pattern and color and the effects of color draping on your skin. It is extremely accurate and reliable, when done properly, focusing on the flattering colors that harmonize with your skin tone.

The Colourflair aim is to concentrate on ensuring that your skin looks as attractive as possible.

This system looks at the facial skin in the way that a plastic surgeon would when deciding how to improve a client's appearance. Scrutinizing lines, wrinkles, blemishes, dark shadows, and other problems, the correct colors are chosen that reduce these issues sometimes as dramatically and with such a transformational effect as a surgical face lift! The real magic is that it can be better than botox because color will give you all the benefits and you can still move your face without having wasted hundreds of pounds.

The four basic families of colors are known as "Seasons" relating to cool Summer and Winter and warm Spring and Autumn. This system simply refers to the characteristics and colors that best describe you and your appearance. As in nature there are many varieties of colors and your seasons appearance has an influence on those around you and the way you feel about yourself.

You as an individual contain a unique blend of the four seasonal possibilities of which usually one will predominate and therefore have the strongest influence on your skin tone, personality and health – your Season. It may be that you have a strong influence from a secondary season that may affect your appearance and personality, which could enable you to wear some colors from your secondary season too.

This book will introduce you to your true colors. You will gain a fascinating insight into the whole field of color as it relates to you. This will have practical and profitable results, which will benefit you for the rest of your life.

This is a must have, self help guide. A gift of knowledge that will transform how you feel about wearing black, and the perfect present for all your girlfriends, mothers, daughters and partners!

SOME CELEBRITY COMMENTS!

Diana Moran Green Goddess (70) on her personal view of dressing in black

Diana is an ex-model and famously adorned our screens as The Green Goddess. She is a beautiful lady and a truly inspirational role model for ageing gracefully. Diana knows how to wear black to best effect, looking stylish and slim without ageing her face. Here she shares her tips with you!

In 2010 age has nothing to do with how you dress – for example jeans and a top can be worn by a woman of any age and still look great. So beware of moving into frump mood just because of your age, and learn to dress for your personality instead!

Whatever your size or shape wearing one block of solid color creates a longer, leaner look, it stops cutting the body in half which makes it appear shorter. But be aware of where your top finishes, especially if you're wearing a sweater with trousers or a skirt because the eye is drawn to where the two meet - which too often is the widest part of the hips!

The solution is to wear either a shorter or a longer top to create a leaner effect. A solid block of black will create a slim, somber silhouette but you may need to give it a "lift" with the addition of color.

Colors are important and help create moods. But, it's imperative to recognize that as we age we lose pigment and color from our skin, our complexion and our hair color changes. Colors, which once suited in our youth, or even 10 years ago, may do nothing for us in maturity. Wearing a flattering color next to the skin is a subtle way of putting color back into an older jaded face without having to use much, if any make-up.

As an amateur artist I use The Color Wheel (an artist's aid) to tell me which colors compliment or clash with another. Ones which sit happily alongside one another, are those directly opposite the other across the wheel. You can see this harmony in nature, and my favourite flower the pansy illustrates it beautifully - purple compliments yellow.

Clothes can affect our mood, so making an effort to dress up a bit makes me feel good (even if nobody else notices!). Layering clothes is not only pretty, but practical too, especially in climate changes, which are created by air conditioning and central heating. When I put an outfit together and have doubts about the effect, I remember what my Mother taught me "when in doubt leave out" and I try a different combination.

As we mature, many older women wear black to be safe. Personally I have to feel on top of the world in order to wear it well, and if I'm feeling low wearing an all black outfit can be a big mistake! For my work in London I find the trick is to add a colorful pashmina, brooch or necklace near my face in a color that really flatters me. When you get it right, a black outfit can look sensational!

The solution is to experiment with inexpensive colorful accessories, flowers, and textures. Mix textures and fabrics – such as a strong black leather jacket over a soft black silk dress.

A little splash of color can lift a black outfit, so being a bit "arty" I enjoy seeing different colors pulling a look together creating unexpected, exciting effects. Be bold, a colorful scarf or startling piece of jewelery need not be expensive but will give interest to a simple black outfit. A trimming or decoration worn near a pretty face will bring attention up to your assets and disguise the body faults lower down!

Use color to the same effect, for example if you have big thighs, wear black on the bottom half and keep your brightest colors to draw attention to your top half. Conversely, a really bright top is not a good idea if you are busty or have a less than flat tummy. The trick here is to wear that little black dress or a black top teamed with black trousers or skirt for a lengthening, slimming effect.

By wearing a pleasing colored jacket over will flatter your skin - but at **the same time** will draw attention **away** from your tubby tummy (which has been disguised by the black top underneath the jacket!)

I lead a very busy life and organize my clothes by color. I have a huge amount of black in my wardrobe - dresses, skirts, trousers and jackets. I would never buy garments in colors just because they are "fashionable" and only wear colors that suit me, lift my spirits and make me feel happy.

I hang all my clothes in color groups – greens (of course), yellows, reds, purples and that large black section! This way I quickly find garments I want and can easily co-ordinate them. It avoids panic buying and the frustration I later feel when I discover I'd already had something similar buried in my wardrobe or drawer for years! So if you're stuck in a style rut, start organizing your wardrobe, keep clearing out and don't hoard. The charity shops are grateful for your cast-offs and you will be helping others less fortunate than yourself.

And finally – look at the shape you're in! Size matters and should not automatically increase with the increase in years! So help yourself look good and feel great by keeping active and eating less in order to enjoy life in your mature years.

Davina Mackail – Author of The Dream Whisperer, on her journey with wearing black

Davina consulted me before her book launch due to all the media appearances that she was about to do. As a stunning blue eyed, blonde, a classic Spring lady, this is how she has adapted to wearing black, which is not in her color range.

"Working with Jules and her approach to the psychology of color through the eyes and personality traits was a revelation to me. I had "my colors done" many years previously and at the time was diagnosed as being able to wear black and white and all the dark, bold colors as the consultant based her analysis on the fact I was blonde, with pale blue eyes and a pale complexion.

At the time I was delighted at not having to eradicate black from my wardrobe yet what I have learnt from Jules has transformed both my wardrobe and the way I look. Those dark colors do not suit me at all and I was shocked at how they aged me and brought my wrinkles to prominence in the mirror during my analysis with her. Now I am learning to wear my true colors, a far lighter, brighter palette.

For my book launch I avoided the ubiquitous black party dress and went for a strong, bright Purple jacket – I'm still reveling in the myriad of compliments I received about how great I looked. This was especially pleasing as many guests were old friends I had not seen for years. I'm also enjoying a new love affair with orange and coral - shades I wouldn't have been seen dead in a few years back. Yet they are shades that suit me perfectly and I feel alive and energized when wearing them.

In fact, although my wardrobe still contains some sexy black items that I am reluctant to part with just yet, since Jules' visit I can't actually persuade myself back into black! That's how radical and profound the shift has been.

I'm thoroughly enjoying shopping within my new color palette and experimenting with other unusual (for me!) colors that I have avoided all my life under the misapprehension that they didn't "suit me". I look better and younger but more importantly I *feel* better in my new colors – they actually give me energy and revitalize my system. I'm just so pleased I discovered this before I got too old to enjoy it!"

I feel incredibly privileged to have had the opportunity to meet and work with women like Janey Lee Grace, Diana Moran and Davina Mackail. By contributing to this book, they have helped to get the message across just how important color is. I have been lucky to encounter many different types of women in my job, from housewives, to managing directors. It is always a joy to see the dramatic and positive affects putting women in their true colors has on their looks and personalities. The right colors can be life changing, and I hope that this book goes some way to changing yours!

CHAPTER TWO

BLACK BEAUTY

How Color Affects Your Face

Growing Old Gracefully

Let's be honest, we all want to look good for as long as possible. Like myself, you may have spent your youth damaging your hair with dodgy dyes and perms, burnt your skin sunbathing to excess and used as many cheap, chemical products you could get your hands on. Suddenly you reach a time where you realize that you have got older and that the damage has started to catch up with you. It is no longer possible to get away with the wrong colored hair and clothing any more! None of us wants to age but as its inevitable, so let's do it gracefully and try and keep looking good for as long as we can.

Your self image is inextricably linked to appearance and is central to your identity. With age comes a changing face, which can have a huge impact when it starts to happen. If feeling good is reliant upon looking good then self image has to change with age in order for women to feel truly happy in their own skin, however wrinkled.

Women today are expected to look fashionable, slim, perfectly groomed and young all of the time, as celebrity role models are idolized in our society for their looks and their lifestyle.

Which fear is greater then? Growing old with fading looks or trying to keep them and possibly ending up looking like someone you don't recognize? It makes sense that if we make our faces look "better", then we will feel more confident inside.

Accepting that beauty and confidence inside and out should

work together, then making the best of your appearance in whatever way suits you is surely the way to lasting contentment.

Cosmetic procedures fell by 12% in the US in 2009, suggesting that the novelty stage is over. Perhaps the extreme make-over shows have given plastic surgery a tacky image, along with media pictures of aging celebrities, who have clearly taken changing their faces too far.

As you age, chemical changes that rob collagen of its solubility and flexibility occur because of oxidation that damages the skin. Treatments and surgery can be expensive, time consuming and often change the look of the face, not to mention are toxic, and a threat to health. One in three women in the UK over 30, uses an anti-ageing product, but Gisele Mir, a cosmetic scientist and founder of MIR Skin Care says "There is no miracle ingredient that will take years off your appearance. The only miracle is that the cosmetics industry has managed to persuade us otherwise for so long."

Skin gradually loses its youthful appearance as you age. It is normally during your mid 30's that the negative effects of ageing on the skin start to appear. Collagen and elastic production starts to slow down which makes the skin thinner, losing its firmness and will result in the tell tales signs of wrinkles and lines. Circulation becomes slower so the cells are not receiving as much oxygen, which means that dead skin cells can remain on the surface of the face giving it a dull look.

Combine these changes with female hormonal fluctuations and this leads to a reduction in sebum production, which means that the skin becomes dryer and can have a more uneven, blotchy look to it.

Some women notice these ageing signs gradually, and for others it can be a sudden onslaught of negatives that appear on the face. Either way, ageing happens to us all.

Making the most of your appearance whatever age is all about maintaining a healthy body and mind, as well as taking the best care of your skin and hair, which in my case has been switching to natural and where-ever possible, organic products.

Feeling good about your image and knowing that you look your best will help in coming to terms with fading looks as you age.

How important it is then to have practical tools that you can use in the fight against anti-ageing. If you knew how powerful the effects of color were up against your skin, it would save you a fortune in the future on buying the wrong outfits, ineffective skin products and huge amounts on cosmetic surgery!

Becoming more beautiful with age is simple if you know how to wear the right colors up against your skin. You could look years younger, not to mention healthier and happier. This alone could give you that longed for self esteem - a well needed boost to your flagging confidence. It is natural, and as cheap or expensive as you want it to be.

Color is key – a tool of knowledge – and understanding what suits your own individual genetic coloring is vital. If black is not in your color range then it will be harmful to your ageing process.

The Ageing Face of Black

So why is black detrimental to the ageing skin? Let me explain.

Black can make a warm skin tone look older because up against the face it reflects and therefore highlights all that is dark; shadows around the chin, lines either side of the mouth, deep grooves between the nose and mouth, forehead lines, dark rings under the eyes. Wrinkles and sunken areas will appear deeper and obviously the older you are the more pronounced this will get.

If you have a warm skin tone black will flatten your complexion, giving it a grey appearance, making you look older, drained and tired. It will take away that golden glow making you appear unhealthy and tired.

Black clothing will also throw a grey overlay onto warm skins because it is out of harmony with them. Dark patches on the face will therefore stand out in the corners of the eyes and around the mouth. Unflattering features will be highlighted and outlined such as a large nose or jaw. The effects are severe and very ageing. Ever noticed that "moustache" effect? That's black for you!

The key is knowing whether you have the pale cool, dramatic skin tone that can wear black well without any of the above negative effects or a warm skin tone that will be aged.

Understanding how to use black is therefore vital to keeping your face looking youthful and healthy.....and its not just black but all dark colors that have black in it like Navy Blue.

If you love wearing black and find this information hard to believe, then do the self help genetic tests in this book so that you can see for yourself whether it ages your face or not.

Wouldn't you rather know?

Now you can look great in black without ageing your face. With the right colors to suit your skin tone, you can continue to wear your favourite black clothing but know how to counteract the negative, ageing and draining effects that black (and other colors with black in them) has.

It is as simple as adding colored accessories to your wardrobe, learning what colors to wear and what make up will bring out the best of your features. Your harmonizing colors will naturally and effectively take years off your face.

Tell all your girlfriends! A way to wear to black and look young and healthy as well as slim and stylish!

Skin Tones

Understanding your skin tone is the one of the keys to knowing what colors really suit you best.

The three pigments of the skin that give you your color are melanin, the brown tones, carotene, the yellow skin tones, and hemoglobin, which gives skin its pink and red hues. One of these pigments may dominate your skin or maybe you have a combination of all three pigments, for example rosy cheeks are a sign of high hemoglobin.

So, which skin tone do you have? Below is a brief summary of cool and warm skin tones broken into the seasonal types. When you have carried out the self help chapters later on in the book, you will find out which genetically inherited skin tone you have.

Cool Skin Tones

These skins have a blue/pink undertone. They can generally be broken down into two seasonal types:

Summer complexions are normally light and rather colorless although occasionally may be slightly darker. This skin never has a "high rosy cheek color" and looks best in pastel shades. Being generally pale and fine textured, these complexions do not tan well and when they do the skin can take on a rather grayish look.

Dark colors, including black are much too strong with these delicate complexions and will highlight any dark, negative things on the skin.

Winter complexions whilst also being cool can be either light or dark and not as translucent as the summer skin. Like cool Summer there is no high color on the skin (not to be mistaken for veins).

Winters have an unusual and often distinctive look to their appearance and whilst pastel shades suit Summers they tend to be too pale for most Winters, who look fabulous in black without showing any signs of darkness on the face.

Warm Skin Tones

These have either yellow/gold or bronze undertones and are split into two seasonal types:

Spring complexions are yellow or gold and they tend to blush easily often with a high rosy cheek color. Spring complexions have a great deal of variety and can have either very fair skin (and often mistaken for the pale Summer complexion but look awful in cool pastels) can be red haired and freckled (do not tan well) or can be dark with skins that generally tan well with a lovely gold color.

Autumns, whilst having similar gold undertones have a more orange skin, with a bronze look to the complexion. This skin tone differs from Spring in that there is never a rosy cheek color.

Warm skins (with whatever hair color) do not look good with black up against the face. It has the negative effect of flattening out the warm skin color and highlighting dark shadows, lines and wrinkles. Basically it ages the face, in some cases more dramatically than others, and these effects worsen with age.

Dark Skin Tones

Darker skinned women with African, West Indian, Asian, Oriental and Latin tones are often able to wear darker shades of color in their clothing and make up, however, it is the pattern and color of the eyes as well as the black draping against the face that will determine who can wear what well. These darker skin tones all show exactly the same effects as lighter tones or black are put up against the face.

Dark skinned women do not automatically fall into the Winter season, and it has been our experience at Colourflair that often these skin tones fall into the warm seasonal palette. Pat says "Generally the darkening of features is the last thing these females want. I have never had anyone of African extraction who was cool and only one Asian who was a Summer".

These are the most common questions I am asked by clients about skin tone:

Does my skin tone change with age?

It is true that our skin will fade as we age, as all our coloring does, but our skin tone remains the same as it is genetic. The key is to use different shades of your own colors, perhaps not as strong or bright as you would have done when you were younger.

The mistake often made by older women with warm skin tones is go into cooler colors when their hair goes grey/white possibly to match it! What they don't realize is that their hair then becomes the focus along with their clothes and not the face. Thus proving that analysis based on hair color alone is not a reliable guide to your underlying skin tone.

What happens when we tan, can we wear different colors?

Sun tanning obviously darkens a warm skin but it does not change our color range. We still have the same skin tones underneath, but in a darker hue. What this means is that stronger, brighter colors that suit you can be worn, and turquoise will always bring out the best tan.

Does health affect our skin tone?

It may well be that a period of bad health affects our skin tone to some degree. How often have you seen someone recovering from the flu who looks positively washed out and pale? I had a client who was finishing a course of chemotherapy from breast cancer whose skin had a grey tinge to it from all the toxins in her system. It is even more important to get the right colors up against the skin when you are ill, to help in your recovery, and to bring out the correct underlying skin tone.

How do cosmetics make a difference?

Make up plays an important role for the complexion at any age, but particularly from age thirty onwards it becomes more important to camouflage the negative aspects that start to appear due to the ageing process. The right color base is essential because the complexion becomes less even as we age. What colors are you using on your face and are they the right tone for your skin or do you need to change to either a cooler or warmer shade?

As the dark shadows, lines, wrinkles and blemishes of age start to show the right colored foundation is key and can be transformational on the ageing skin. It also becomes more important to accentuate your good features, and the right colored blusher and eye make up will ensure harmony and a natural look that will make you look younger and healthier.

It's not just older women that benefit from understanding the basic color of their complexion. Teenage girls starting to wear make up benefit hugely from knowing whether their base should be more yellow, orange or pink. It helps them to avoid years of make up mistakes and the wrong colored eye shadow! Features can be enhanced dramatically by using the correct colors on the right skin tone, so starting early will always be beneficial in the long run.

A full range of cool and warm seasonal colors are discussed further in the self help chapters of this book once you have discovered your own personal color schemes.

CHAPTER THREE

BLACK BACKGROUND

Historical Influences

You have got to this chapter and are probably wondering what history has to do with your colors? Let's be honest, history only really gets interesting when it relates directly to you as an individual. Why is the color black part of your wardrobe and what is its association with death and gloom? Why is color analysis important and where did it come from? Can colors really affect your health and well being? This chapter is directly related to you, because it is a fascinating insight into why you wear black today. It provides a background of factual information on the history of black in fashion, color analysis and in healing.

Throughout history, for cultural and religious reasons black has symbolized many things; death, mourning, poverty and power. We have been conditioned to wear black with fashion trends spearheading how to wear it, often related to economic situations. Over the past two years since the recession began, the media and high street have focused very much on black in fashion, which has coincided with the financial depression and uncertainly.

Black has a dark side, what with black magic and witches' hats and things that go bump in the night. It's interesting to look at where this all began and how black has become so popular in our modern times. Somewhere in your subconscious it will have influenced your feelings about black.

IN FASHION

In the church it was as early as the fifth century that religious figures were wearing black as a symbol of the mourning of Christ. Their clothing was worn as religious symbolism with the Roman collar for obedience; the sash or cincture around the waist, chastity; and the color black, poverty. For priests, black did not just represent mourning but dying, resurrecting and serving the Lord as well as giving witness of the Kingdom yet to come.

The church had incredibly strict dress rules and the priests black cassocks had to be correctly worn at the right length or penalties were enforced upon them. Whilst Catholic dress regulations have become more relaxed over the ages, the color black has remained a religious symbol of belief and service to the church, as still worn today by priests and nuns.

Black took on a powerful and authoritative status of its own during the fifteenth and sixteenth centuries when men in Parliament and the Court of the King made it fashionable. During the seventeenth century the prosperous Dutch also wore black during a period of great wealth in the Netherlands. Only the wealthy and well connected could afford to wear black clothes as they were expensive due to the lack of appropriate dyes available, so black clothing lost its humble image.

In the nineteenth century the romantic poets and men of status became known as "dandies" representing the image of the perfect gentleman, and thus black became "the" color for men to be seen in. Black was also adopted as attire for the working merchant classes who wore it conservatively to indicate economic stability during that period. It was a time when clerics, teachers, judges, medics and domestics all started wearing black.

During the nineteenth century black become known as the "straightforward color of death". Queen Victoria had a rather "melancholic" childhood as she was raised in near isolation, so was left devastated when her husband Prince Albert died.

She grieved in black for the remainder of her life, thus setting a precedent for other widows of that time. Black therefore came to indicate deep sorrow and profound grief and mourning, which again became popular during World War 1.

Late that century The Black Tie emerged for eveningwear, which was a formal dress code for men consisting of black jacket and trousers, bow tie and often cummerbund and waistcoat. Women were expected to wear long, smart dresses.

French designer Coco Chanel revolutionized haute couture fashion in the 1920's and 30's by introducing a simple chic, unstructured black shift dress. "The Little Black Dress" became famous when worn by Audrey Hepburn in the 1961 film Breakfast at Tiffany's and still remains a fashion staple in most women's wardrobes today.

Wallis Simpson, Duchess of Windsor, owned several LBD's and was quoted as saying "when a little black dress is right there is nothing else to wear in its place".

Hollywood women started wearing black when black and white television first become popular and it was thanks to Christian Dior who gave the little black dress an air of danger and drama. Celebrities are now often seen on the red carpet showcasing the drama and glamour of black.

The 1960's saw the emergence of the punk culture in America which filtered through to the UK a decade or so later. Their dress code included black bin liners that were ripped up, with the added embellishment of safety pins, studs and chains. The aim was to create an image of rebellion, along with the desire to shock the general public with their antisocial behavior.

The need to appear menacing to others is often behind these black fashions; as black is the total absorption of color it provides a psychological barrier and protection from society, so that as a color black became a statement for deeper psychological issues. Black is also often worn during demonstrations against political systems as it is seen as anarchic.

Black is also worn to symbolize authority in society, in the police force, in the church, and our legal system. For the lawyers and judges black wields power as it does for policemen and women and it also provides protection for them.

When we go back through the ages and look at how we associate black with historical events we can see how it has affected our culture and religion today.

IN COLOUR ANALYSIS

Personal color analysis is becoming more and more widely understood. As the physiological and psychological effects of color are central to your well being and to the way you present yourself, it is also vital to your health, beauty and self confidence. Understanding that the connection between the colors you are most attracted to can also reflect your personal coloring and temperament. When coupled with the patterns in your eyes this is incredibly valuable in gaining appreciation of how to blend this knowledge to the best effect.

Where did it all begin?

The great philosopher Aristotle (384BC-322BC) had a theory that has formed the basis of color work for over 2000 years. His view was that the two primary colors were white and black i.e. light and dark, and that all colors were derived from one of 4 elements; air, water, earth and fire. He also believed that if you stared at black or into darkness that blue was the first color to appear. Likewise if you looked at sunlight then yellow was the first color. Thus he believed the true primary colors after black and white were blue and yellow.

The English scientist Isaac Newton (1642-1727) discovered that the colors of the spectrum were all contained in pure light. He shone white light through a triangular prism whereby the different wavelengths refracted at different angles through sunlight giving us the "rainbow" effect. Newton's Theory of Color was based on the fact that objects did not generate colors themselves, rather they interacted with already colored light.

In 1810 the German philosopher Johann Wolfgang von Goethe published his Theory of Colors. Whilst he made an exhaustive study of color he did not link his theories with clothing colors or their influence on the face.

Historically, it was the Frenchman Michel Eugene Chevreul (1786-1889) who was the first so called "color consultant". As director of a well-known tapestry firm he noticed when looking at colors how they interacted differently when placed side by side compared to when viewed alone. This led him to discover that when the eye looks at a certain color it demands that the opposite or contrasting color on the color wheel is seen i.e. when looking at red, the eye generates green – what we now call, its complimentary color.

Chevreul wrote a book about his findings called De la Loi de Contraste Simultane des Couleurs (Of the Law of Simultaneous Contrast of Colors). In the book he devoted a chapter to the subject of colors worn against the face, including hair color, and determined that these would affect the appearance of the skins color.

The Bauhaus school was founded in 1919, where many influential artists were brought together. One of these was the Swiss expressionist painter Johannes Itten (1888-1967). Whilst teaching painting, he noticed that when his students were given identical studies, some opted for warm colors that matched their own warm coloring, whilst others chose cool colors to match their cool coloring. This suggested to him that most people fundamentally knew the colors they are most comfortable with.

Thus the basis of Itten's theory was that colors have either a blue based undertone or a yellow one, and this formed the basic foundation of color analysis that we use today. His was the first breakthrough in discovering color pallets for people.

The American Robert Dorr went on to create the Color Key System in 1938 by dividing colors into cool and warm. This became the start of personal color analysis.

His suggestion was that you chose the colored fan that you preferred, and then made all your choices from that range, as they were all in harmony with each other as well as the individuals coloring. Summer and Winter's cool colors could be found in Key 1, and Spring and Autumns warm colors in Key 2. this was widely used in the 1940's and became a major influence in designing colors in all its aspects.

What is Color?

You process color in the right side of your brain, which is your intuitive side, and shape in your left side, which is the male and intellect. This means that in order to understand how color affects you, you will have to combine your intellect and also the feminine side of your emotions. True knowledge of the effect of colors can only really be achieved by your own experiences of them. Each day you may feel the need for a different color because your emotions permanently change and you will have different color requirements to help keep you in a healthy balance.

Your eyes see color as light. It is then the retina, which converts these light vibrations into electrical impulses. These get fed into the hypothalamus gland in the brain, which in turn affects your hormonal system, which is why in winter and countries that experience periods that lack daylight there is a tendency for depression. Your body needs light. Different colored wavelengths need different adjustments in the eyes, with red having the longest wavelength and therefore needing the most adjustment, and green requiring no adjustment.

Your own personal feelings about color will differ from the next person, as color is subjective to each individual. The girl that hates green because she had to wear it as a school uniform will almost certainly have trouble wearing it again. Each individual's reaction to color will depend on personality as well as circumstances.

Colors are everywhere, because everything has a color. In nature it is abundant and supports us throughout the year.

In Spring the colors are clear and bright and the green shades in nature are tinged with yellow undertones. The sun starts to reflect its light on everything giving the landscape a warmth and brightness. Flowers and foliage become vibrant with bright red tulips and yellow daffodils in abundance.

In Summer the colors become faded and dusky due to the suns rays, and hues become muted with blue undertones. Baby blues and pale pinks are everywhere and roses and lavender bloom.

In Autumn the rich earthy harmonious tones of golden based colors emerge, oranges, mustards, shades of brown and olive greens, teal blues and rust that have such wonderfully warm dramatic shades.

In Winter colors become icy and clear, with blue undertones. The landscape becomes very black and white and it is a time of hibernation and minimalism.

So, the psychology of color relates personality types to the four seasons, and therefore having your own colors around you will vibrate with you individually and on an energetic level, bringing happiness and harmony into your life. Choosing to live and wear colors that suit you personally is not about what color is fashionable, but what color makes you look and feel great when you surround yourself with it.

THE COLOUR WHEEL

As seen on the front cover of the book, the color wheel gives you an idea of how colors separate into cool and warm shades starting with yellow through to violet-red being seen as warm with red-orange the warmest and from yellow-green to violet as cold, with blue-green the coldest. Spring/Autumn colors are termed warm, and Summer/Winter cool.

Green, due its combination of both cool blue and warm yellow is understandably a flexible color in terms of skin tone. When you add black it becomes a winter, cool color, and with white a summer, pastel one. Add more yellow to brighten it up for springs warm tones, and with red it becomes autumn green.

Turquoise is THE most flexible color for all skin tones but adding even small amounts of color can change its hue to be more flattering for different skins. Warm tones will veer towards teal, and cool tones, aqua. Turquoise is also the best color to wear if you want to enhance your tan!

Primary red crosses over between Spring and Winter - with more yellow it becomes warmer whereas adding blue it becomes cooler.

The Spectrum represents all the colors contained in the rainbow; red, orange, yellow, green, blue and indigo. **Color Hues** are colors of the spectrum, and it is that which distinguishes one color from another. **Primary Colors** are basic colors that are not a mixture of other colors; red, yellow and blue. All colors are created with these three primaries combined with black and white.

Tints and Shades - a color added to white is a tint and added to black a shade. **Intermediate Colors** are mixed from two primaries in unequal amounts i.e. yellow-orange, blue-green. **Complementary Colors** sit opposite each other on the color wheel i.e. red and green, blue and orange.

IN HEALING

Color affects your life in many ways and used positively can have a profound healing benefit to you, physically and emotionally. You can express yourself through the colors that you wear and use them in a powerful way to communicate with others. Black, grey and brown are not colors that are generally used in healing as they are too dense and heavy and therefore not suitable for use in healing therapies.

The Research

The Pythagoreans in 500bc became aware of vital energy and its healing powers in the form of light. They named this healing energy "mumia". The mathematician Johannes Baptist Van Helmonts in the 17th century suggested that pure vital energy penetrates and supports every material thing including our physical bodies. He claimed that cures could be found in magnetic treatments using "mumia".

In ancient Egypt special diagnostic rooms in temples were erected where sunlight shining into them was refracted into colors of the spectrum. Sick patients were then placed inside these special healing rooms and flooded with the appropriate colors assigned to their illness. The early Greeks carried out similar practices by exposing sick people to the sun.

In ancient India minerals and colored gemstones were used for healing. The revival of color therapy in the eleventh century by the Persian physician Avicenna, noted that red increased blood pressure and blue lowered it. The Russian Scientist S.V. Krakov went on to prove Avicenna's theory about the effects of red and blue on the body.

Scientists have continued over time to research the aura and in the 18th century a German Mathematician Gottfied Wilhelm Leibritz believed that everyone was interconnected energetically. In the 1800's German scientist Baron Karl Von Reichenbach conducted experiments to prove that certain people were sensitive to seeing colors around living beings.

In the early 1900's, light therapy was brought to the fore when Niels Finsen won the Nobel prize for successful cure of skin tuberculosis using light and color. Since then medical science has found light helps to cure skin conditions, burns and wounds and is also a great pain reliever.

In 1908 Dr Walter Kilner observed the aura of his medical patients through colored screens and was able to describe how the inner aura followed body contours and the outer aura was longer and ovoid. His discovery was a breakthrough as it proved that most of us can see auras by simply changing the focus of our eyes.

One of the biggest breakthroughs in recent times on energy photography was in 1939 by Semyon Kirlian who accidentally discovered that if an object on a photographic plate was connected to a source of high voltage then small corona discharges create an image on that plate. He claimed that these images showed the aura around a living being, and went on to carry out many experiments to prove his theories.

In the early 1980's biologist and scientist Harry Oldfield discovered that diseased states manifest first in the body's energy field and went on to develop methods to treat energy imbalances; a system called Electro Crystal Therapy (ECT).

Using microchip technology he developed a scanner, called a Polycontract Interference Photography (PIP), which could provide a real time, moving image of the energy field. He then devised a computer programme that would analyze the different light intensities being reflected from the scanned person or object. This gave a simple and accurate assessment of the energy imbalances, which provided the trained eye with details of the state of health and well being of the scanned individual.

This is what Harry says about black:

"This is not really a color but a total absence of any light. A surface is black when it absorbs all light falling on it and does not itself emit light. In our PIP Reality system filter which is based on investigations on what some clairvoyants see, black has been allocated the color to denote areas of absence of light and sometimes indicates a lack of life force. It can also be evidence above the head of cases of severe depression".

Energy, the Aura and Color Therapy

Everything in our world vibrates with energy; people, animals, trees, plants and all living beings. As the amazing Russian healer Alla Svirinskaya says in her book Energy Secrets "the very first principle of good health is healthy energy. If your energy is healthy, not only will your body be healthy but your life will be too. The easiest way to understand the principles of the energy that fuels our lives and our beings is to adopt and adapt some of the basic tenets of Eastern philosophy. This claims that human beings consist of a physical body and seven subtle energy bodies. The aura is not one spiritual body but actually the combined seven bodies. Each of these bodies is different and distinct and each has clearly defined functions. They are inter-connected and dependent on each other and our good health relies on the good health of each and every one of them".

Ever since time began the aura or energy field has been documented as rays of light coming off the body. In religion it has been depicted as the image of a halo, and in Hindu and Buddhist teachings this related to the seven chakras (wheels) or energy centers of the body. These colored energy centers of red, orange, yellow, green, blue, indigo and purple are in the subtle body surrounding your physical one. They do not include black.

The chakras keep you well when balanced, but when they get out of balance all kind of emotional and physical problems can start to manifest. By bringing your minds and bodies into harmony, you can restore your well being and in this way color acts as a powerful remedy.

Your aura of light and color reflect your health and well being. You radiate with light when well and when feeling "off color" the aura colors appears drab and dull. These bright clear colors of health can become muddy when negative emotions such as greed and fear are felt strongly or during a period of illness.

You may sometimes be drawn to colors that are actually in your own aura and one color may predominate or there may be lots of different ones. If you constantly wear colors that are not in harmony with your energy field and personality, you wont feel at your best and your looks will most definitely suffer as a result.

Your particular need of a color may well be related to an area of your body that needs healing. As colors affect the entire energy field, the ones that you wear a lot will become part of your aura as they remain there even after you have removed the colored clothing. So if you wear a lot of black you are constantly draining your energy field of color.

Ever wondered why you are drawn to a particular color one day and a different one the next? Wearing colors that you are attracted to at a certain time for either emotional or physical reasons will give you a psychological boost, making you feel good because you will be releasing endorphins, which in turn strengthens your immune system.

Alison Standish (no relation!) is a color therapist and this is what she says about healing with colors and black. "Color therapy uses both ancient and modern technologies to combine as a treatment for the body to allow the absorption of certain colors for certain ailments. Our electromagnetic field or Aura gives bio readings on how we are feeling and whether we have any dis-ease. Colors can then be applied to the body to help support and cure this dis-ease before it becomes a physical disease.

The eyes only use 25% of the color they receive for seeing and that the remaining 75% is absorbed in the body to help support the nervous and immune system. In color therapy black represents respite and a chance to get away from unwanted attention. I never use the color on its own and very rarely use it in a color treatment.

Black stones in treatments, such as hematite, tourmaline and smoky quartz are sometimes placed under the bed as a way of connecting the client to the earth energies and keeping the client grounded. It can allow access to hidden pain and find hidden skills within us but as I am always using other colors, there is a balance so that black never becomes overpowering. As the practitioner, I usually wear black or white so that the client does not absorb any additional colors other than the colors used in the treatment. This also allows my energies to be preserved, keeps me 'earthed' and not deplete me during the treatments".

As an individual your needs will be personal to you. Color can be used as a healing tool in many ways, by simply experiencing sunlight and being surrounded by nature. Sometimes just looking at beautiful spring flowers can be enough to brighten your spirits.

The best way to use color for your own healing good, is to wear your true colors, the ones that make you smile when you see yourself, the ones that people comment on when they see you, and the ones that support you emotionally each and every day.

You have the power to bring harmony into your own life. Particularly when experiencing difficult situations, color can be very beneficial in promoting your health and sense of well being. Color vibrations are absorbed through your eyes and your skin as well as through your aura so that you have the power within to restore and revitalize your body and your emotions.

Discovering your true colors can change your life!

CHAPTER FOUR

THE PSYCHOLOGY OF BLACK
Your Relationship with Color

Since time began men have wondered what makes women tick! The female psyche when it comes to appearance and looking good is both complex and simple. Complex because there can be so many emotional reasons why particular outfits and colors are chosen. Simple because most women really just want to look their best; slim and attractive, young and healthy. No wonder men are confused!

It is important to understand that colors have powerful effects on your personality and your emotions because they influence you through your eyesight and skin. This is why wearing the right colors to match your personality and genetic coloring is vital for your well being and self confidence. There will be colors that support you psychologically and emotionally, and others that suppress your true nature.

Dr. Victoria Galbraith of Galbraith Consultancy, a Chartered Counseling Psychologist, Life Coach and Senior Lecturer provides us with a fascinating insight into black:

"The color black has great psychological and symbolic meaning. Black is regularly associated with darkness of mind and is always contrasted with lightness of spirit. As well as being an analogy, the color black is also reflected in what a person does and in the creativity that emanates from them. My psychotherapy clients often refer to feeling as though they are in a 'black hole' and wanting to see the 'light at the end of the tunnel'.

When people are feeling low, vulnerable or out of control, they may project how they are feeling into a color...often this color is black! They may draw or paint with black hues...and this can happen from a very early age.

Time and time again, the shade that reflects the sadness experienced is black. And this reflection of mood can translate in a much more subtle way by extending to the colors we wear. Of course, black has become synonymous with sadness...we only need to look at how grieving friends and relatives choose to wear black for a funeral, both as a sign of respect but also as a reflection of feeling.

I have known clients who may choose to respect the wishes of a deceased friend or relative by wearing their choice of vibrant colors to a funeral to "celebrate their life" but their first preference would always be to wear black. They feel sadness and loss...and they feel the need to project this feeling through their clothes.

So, if you are a black wearer...rather than relying on the color black to fulfill this 'esteem' function through the power, safety or sexiness you feel it gives you, try to gain this feel good factor from within. When you do, it will be portrayed into the way that you communicate with others, both verbally and through your body language; it will affect your poise, stature and presence...and more importantly, it will affect how others relate to you which in turn will affect how you see yourself!"

Philippa Merivale author of "Rescued by Angels" and "The Wizdom of Oz" feels that black should be explored as a place to find your own dark and inner emotions.

"Only when we feel safe do we dare to even look at our own shady places. The outside always reflects the inside, in one way or another, so make a good friend of the outer black – the dress that makes you feel good enough to be nice to yourself – and you can start making friends with what's inside as well. Not just the pretty bits, but all of it.

Dare to dig a little, beneath the safe protection of your dusky robes, and in that inner darkness, yes, you will doubtless find some of the pesky thoughts and characteristics that have not served your very best interests; but here, concealed in the shadows, are skills and talents that you would never have dreamed could be your very own.

And so you will find that you are an amazing, magnificent, wonderful woman with gifts that surpass anything that has ever been achieved on the catwalk.

Now that is *real* power".

It is true to say that women wear black for many different psychological reasons. It's slimming, easy to put together, a safe option, protective, stylish and smart, and hopefully this chapter will provide you with an insight into the many reasons why you might wear black.

The Color Concept
Looking at how the great philosophers in history related color to personality and its effects on our present day life is both fascinating and revealing. Also, understanding how the four temperaments and colors physically affect you will highlight what impact they have psychologically on your life.

Johanne Wolfgang Goethe, was the first philosopher and writer of the late 18th century to study the psychological effects of color. He believed that color had an immediate effect on emotions and in 1810 published his book the "Theory of Colors". Carl Jung also used symbolism through color and encouraged his patients to paint and express their deep subconscious issues through color.

In the early 20th century Max Luscher, a professor of psychology at Basle University measured people's preferences for chosen colors and diagnosed and treated physical and psychological conditions.

He devised the Luscher color test, a tool for measuring psychophysical states based on color. He believed that colors have an emotional value and that personality traits are revealed through each individual's color preference.

The American art historian Faber Birren (1900-1988) probably wrote more books on color than anyone else. In his book "Color Psychology And Color Therapy: A Factual Study Of The Influence Of Color On Human Life" he provides us with much credible information about the link between psychology and color.

Dr Kurt Goldstein (1878-1965) a German neurologist and psychiatrist worked with brain injured soldiers in World War I who discovered that color not only affects our entire being but according to his studies, various mental conditions and psychological states respond to color in different ways.

To support his findings he wrote about a woman who had a cerebella disease that meant she fell and walked unsteadily. Interestingly, when she wore a red dress her symptoms got worse, unlike green and blue clothing which had the opposite effect and restored her balance. This suggested that the human organism is disturbed far more by red than it is by green and blue.

Experimental evidence of the effect of pure red shows that it stimulates the nervous system and temporarily increases the metabolic rate through releasing the hormone adrenaline. Blue on the other hand has the ability to calm the nervous system as it circulates the relaxing hormone, oxytocin.

Cool tones have been best administered where routine and monotonous tasks are performed, such as in offices or factories. Warm tones appear to be more suitable to living areas and restaurants where things are likely to seem longer/bigger under warm lights and shorter/smaller under cool ones.

Early in the twentieth century, the value of color conditioning was accepted in hospitals and schools to increase production and to cut down on accidents.

The physician Felix Deutsch's research showed peoples' reactions to color were either repressing or inspiring and in bright, harmonious environments we will find our moods lifting. This then will have a physical affect, improving blood pressure and strengthening the nervous system. Color helps us when we have a predilection for it. Extroverts tend to choose red, while introverts favor blue. This also seems to correlate with brunettes preferring red and blondes blue.

Sunlight (or lack of it) seems to be an important factor when deciding on color preferences. Where sunlight is abundant there is a preference for warm, vivid hues. In areas of less light there it is for cooler, softer shades. Red-sighted nations like the Latinos with their dark eyes, hair and complexions tend to prefer red and warm hues whereas Scandinavian blonds are often green or blue eyed, with pale hair and complexion and prefer the blues and greens.

The Temperaments and Black
It is fascinating to realize that there is indeed a strong connection between your genetically inherited coloring and your basic temperament. This underlying theory was first established by Hippocrates over 2,000 years ago.

He believed that the human body was made up of the four elements of air, water, fire and earth and that corresponding with these were four vital bodily substances or "Humors"; blood, phlegm, yellow bile and black bile. If one of these substances was dominant over the others then this would affect the appearance and the temperament of the individual.

The Sanguine (Spring) temperament had a preponderance of blood. We can see this in the high color often noted in this skin tone and can be seen as blushing or red veins. The Phlegmatic (Summer) temperament had a preponderance of phlegm. The pallor is noted in this skin tone as pale fluid.

The Choleric (Autumn) temperament had a preponderance of yellow bile. This relates to the liver and shades of mustard, which only truly suits the Choleric type. The Melancholic (Winter) temperament had a preponderance of black bile. These skin tones are able to absorb the color black without graying the face.

The early Greek physician Claudius Galen in the 2nd Century went on to develop the four basic temperaments that we use today. He set in motion a systemized method for the study of medicine, developed by others and valued by many.

Each of the four main temperament types has important qualities and a difficult period in your life may activate a part of your personality that you didn't know existed. Any trauma or illness may depress you and bring out the melancholic in your temperament and you may therefore find yourself wearing black clothing as a means of coping with the situation.

The colors that match your temperament are the ones that will be in harmony with the essence of your personality and will give you more energy as well as make you look better. It may be that you have temperament combinations, be very outgoing with a sanguine/choleric mix or be more introverted with a sanguine/phlegmatic combination. In order to find out more about your personality traits, fill out the questionnaire in the self help chapter of this book.

WHY WOMEN WEAR BLACK

Most women love to wear black. In my work I have seen many women dressed in it. Suggesting that they never wear it again can be totally counter productive and sends some into a complete state of panic. However, when I show women how negative it can be against their faces, some will vow never to buy it again, whilst others want to be shown how they can continue to wear it, without ageing themselves.

There are of course many ways that women can continue to have it as a mainstay in their wardrobe once they have learnt how to combine it with the right colors, they can significantly improve the condition and look of the skin.

Black is often seen as a mysterious contradiction: both annihilating, which women often want so they don't stand out in a crowd, and at the same time slimming. A simple yet sophisticated statement, it is often considered the best bet, a safe option because it covers everything.

A lot of women do believe that black is THE best color for all occasions. Whilst there are a vast amount of flattering alternatives to black, one of the problems that women face is that so many items of clothing in the High Street are black. Why is this? The answer is because it sells because women believe it's the fashionable color to be seen in, particularly during the colder months. If women started to show a demand for other flattering colors over the autumn/winter period then almost certainly the retailers and fashion houses would offer a more diverse range.

There is also the misconception that as you get older, you should become more staid with your colors and less "bright". I have seen many women going into their 50's and 60's doing this and simply ending up feeling depressed because they look so gloomy and funereal. Wearing the right colors that suit you can keep you looking younger for much longer.

So, why do women wear black – where do we begin? In my experience I have come across 5 main categories that into which most women will fall. Read through the following and see whether you fit into one or more of them!

1. It is Slimming

"When I'm having a fat day, its straight to the black jacket" (Joan Collins)

Its hard to believe Joan Collins ever having a "fat day" and sadly for most of us warm skinned ladies we don't share her striking cool looks that enable us to look dynamite in black either. Joan's idea of instant glamour for everyone is to wear black, particularly polo necks – unfortunately this just encourages women to look like Morticia from the Adams family, only older.

So why is it that so many women reach for the black outfit first thing in the morning after looking in the mirror and "feeling fat". What is it about black that makes us believe it will instantly take off two dress sizes and make us invisible? This is the nature of our strongly held belief system drummed into us by the media, models, designers and the high street retailers. How can they all be wrong?

Ok, so the reality is that black is only truly slimming if its in your color range. Whilst there are other dark colors that will do the job just as well, if not better, convincing women not to wear black with a weight issue will not work for the majority.

Sandra is a size 16 and she feels "being overweight I find that wearing colors just highlight my lumpy bits, and black camouflages my body and doesn't draw attention to my size. I definitely use black to hide behind and hope that I wont stand out and be noticed. However, I do know that it doesn't flatter me to wear black close to my face."

Colourflair founder Pat Scott Vincent says:

"I was wearing a new cream home made silk suit not in a slimming style, gathered skirt, for goodness sake. Went to a function where everyone thought I had lost weight, which I knew I had not. On leaving a male friend came out to tell me how great and slim I was looking. I was so taken aback, I wore it to my first radio broadcast for confidence.

For years overweight women have been told that they will look slimmer in dark colors. This is because of the optical illusions created by color with brighter, lighter and warmer colors appearing closer when compared to duller, darker and colder colors.

However the truth is that if the dark color you are wearing is not in your range you may well look heavier than in one of your own brighter or lighter shades. Overweight Winters will look marvelous in all over black and navy but sadly for other seasonal types these colors may indeed add weight. Using your own color palette close to your face will create a strong vertical line, which is of benefit. When colors from the same family blend into each other this causes the eye to slide over them and is therefore more slimming"!

The key is to know what colors to wear for maximum effect on your own personal body shape. The general color rule is to use stronger, brighter colors on your best body areas to make them more noticeable/larger. Bright and light colors should run up and down your middle with darker ones on the outside for a slimming effect. Use duller, darker colors on badly proportioned or bigger areas to camouflage and make them appear smaller.

Women come in all shapes and sizes and each of these types has a beauty of her own. As a stylish woman you can enhance and capitalize on your natural body type by using clothing that is harmonious and complementary to your shape and your coloring.

As black highlights all the negatives on the face, particularly as we age, what's the point in looking slimmer if your face looks years older? It is possible for you to look slimmer and younger at the same time, and this book will show you how.

2. It is Easy and Functional

A lot of women wear black because it's easy to co-ordinate – get up in the morning, open the wardrobe "what to wear"? For the office black is functional, practical and professional. However, its also very severe, and depending on your job can make you appear unapproachable.

When it comes to the cocktail party, or even the office, black is in charge, and it's hardly surprising. Glamour aside, black bestows on the wearer an aura of authority and power. Never mind how you feel inside, put on the black suit and any vulnerable interior is instantly covered up, leaving you to get on with your day's work (or play) undisturbed by inner demons.

I have had several clients who were teachers and wore black suits and jackets to school, as they wanted respect from their pupils. This can be very effective for first impressions i.e. walking into a classroom or dealing with a disciplinary situation. Children, however, relate to color very positively.

I was able to show these women that it was possible to wear black to gain respect and also combine it with a color that suited them to help encourage communication with the kids.

If you don't work but still wear black as part of your daily routine, try wearing black basics i.e. trousers or skirts with a colored top – you will be amazed at how much more energy you have, and how much better you will feel every time you look in the mirror because your face will look healthier and younger!

It doesn't cost much to make small changes. T-shirts and tops in colors can be bought on a budget whilst you get used to intro-ducing colors into your wardrobe.

You will feel so much better when you open your wardrobe in the morning to a rainbow of color rather than a depressing rail of black!

3. It is Safe

Leslie is in her 50's and wears black because she feels "safe" in it. An attractive lady who has kept her looks feels that she is "put together" in black, and no-one will judge her appearance because "black is what it is – simple and safe".

Wearing black will ensure you mingle with the crowd. You

won't stand out at a party because the majority of the other women there will also be in black too! It's obvious that if you wear a colored dress you are more likely to get noticed. If you do not want to get some attention and compliments that will boost your self confidence, then play it safe in black. It is emotionally comfortable and will obviously suit the more reserved, introverted women amongst you, but your face does not have to suffer for the sake of being safe.

Dr Victoria Galbraith says "For those who lack confidence, wearing black can assist them with feeling the power, control, sexiness or indeed status that they may crave. However, this communicates something about the person...it implies that they are not at ease with themselves.

It can suggest that they need the security of such a powerful color to have the desired effect on others; and to portray what they indeed wish was a more genuine or natural characteristic e.g. they want to appear powerful because in reality, they feel powerless.

They lack self-esteem so they need the black garments in order to gain esteem from others. But if such people continually wear black it can create a false sense of security, and may contribute to prolonging the belief that they *need* to continue wearing black due to the 'feel good' factor they experience as well as the power they assume it promises them.

Unfortunately, this is just an association – others will react to the black-wearer in a particular way based on the message that their black clothing emanates rather than what the person emanates. Therefore, rather than being reliant on black, a much more ideal situation would be to feel and experience self-esteem from within; a self-esteem that is not dependent on how others see them".

The real Winter, cool coloring will stand out in black, and she will turns heads when she walks in the door. This is because her striking and unusual looks; skin tone, hair and features will all work in harmony with black. However, if you have a warm skin you may well stand out in black for all the wrong reasons. Sadly looking older may be one of them.

Ok, so you're not about to ditch your LBD. There are ways to wear black safely without ageing the face dramatically, so keep reading and you will learn how.

4. It is Protective during Trauma and Illness

When faced with emotional trauma and distress from life changing events such as death, divorce, or a major illness the tendency is to hide from the world until you feel better. The best color for protection from the outside world during these troubled times is black.

During dark periods of mourning or emotional and physical distress black can provide necessary cover - a protection and a shield. It is important that one is allowed periods of grief and introversion when needed and black can play a part during these times.

However, wearing black can become a habit, and eventually stop one from progressing out of the dark periods and recovering.

This is Rachel's story:

"Most of the time, I dip into my black wardrobe once or twice a week when wanting to create an *instant*, smart, classy, classic, ageless look. In black, I don't have to worry about *getting it right*, and can just focus on enjoying myself!

However, in tough times like around my divorce, black stops being my smart, go anywhere, all guns firing uniform and becomes my refuge. It stops being a once or twice a week wear and becomes my permanent color of choice. At such times, I find black very reassuring.

It has an honesty and authenticity to it in mirroring my internal world. I find myself temporarily abandoning flamboyant accessories, instead taking comfort in the ageing, draining qualities of wearing unremitting black! I'm in my cave, resting, recuperating, licking my wounds.

The message is clear – I'm feeling fragile, please handle with care. The more wane I look, the better! I want the world, or at least my girl friends, to know exactly how I feel. The confident, exuberant me is on hold, that is until the mourning is over and I feel ready to re-embrace color and for black to once again fall back into being my smart, classy, perfect companion, fit for all social occasions".

A lady with cancer came to see me having been through several years of treatment. As a result she had lost her hair, which had grown back a different color and texture. She had also put on weight due to the drugs, and lost her skin color. In short, her self confidence was in pieces.

During her illness she had reverted to black and other dark colors. Not surprisingly she was trying desperately to cover up her body as well as her emotional distress.

Having finished her treatment she was very keen to start looking better but did not know where to begin. She decided to have a color consultation, and after showing her how much healthier she looked with the right colored make up and clothes up against her face, she was thrilled. As we lifted off the dark colors and replaced them with her shades of blues, reds and orange I watched her smile light up her face and literally melt away the years of pain.

A week later she contacted me to say how much happier she felt as so many people had complimented her on how well she looked. After so much illness this finally made her realize that there was hope, and she could look attractive again.

Depression is a terrible illness and when I had a client come to me dressed head to toe in black/navy blue and feeling really low due to several life changing events I hoped that color would be able to help her. She was a singer but hadn't had much success up to that point, was single and lived alone. She admitted that she dressed in dark colors because she had an introverted side and liked "hiding".

When we looked at her personality questionnaire I understood why she had found herself going into such dark, drab colors. She had a light golden skin tone with blonde hair, and clear patterned green eyes, and was absolutely bowled over when she saw how great bright, clear, warm colors looked up against her face.

Changing from her habit of dark colors was tough particularly as her emotional life was suffering. She bought small amounts of colored tops that were inexpensive just to make sure she liked them. I had an email a few months later to say how much happier she felt since wearing some bright colors, and she had noticed how much better her skin looked every time she saw herself. She is now married and was nominated for a music Grammy award last year.

Finding your true colors will have a powerful and positive affect on your emotions, whatever situation you may find yourself in, both now or in the future.

5. It is Sexy, Stylish and Smart

That little black dress makes you feel put together, composed and focused. It mysteriously hides what you are thinking and feeling, thus giving it a sexy feel because it gives way to male fantasies and imaginations. So far so good?

Whilst this is all true of the LBD, did you know that men actually react far more passionately to red as a color than black? Red physically raises blood pressure and that is why as a color it is constantly linked to romance and love!

Being sexy comes from an inner confidence. Wearing clothing that makes you feel good about yourself will instantly give you increased confidence, and make you feel sexier whether it is black, or any other color. Wouldn't you feel even better if you knew that the color you wore not only made your figure look great but your face younger and healthier too? If black makes you feel sexy then make sure you are wearing it well, and not unknowingly ageing your face at the same time.

There is no doubt that a black tie event creates a classic and formal evening look that renders most people smart and chic. The little black dress (short or long) and black suits are fashion classics, but only those with true cool coloring will wear these outfits with real sexiness and style as they are ones who naturally harmonize with black and white.

If you want to continue to wear your LBD and other black outfits because they make you fell sexy and stylish, there is a way to look classic but not age your face. The following chapters in this book will help you to learn how this can be done, effortlessly and stylishly!

CHAPTER FIVE

DO YOU HAVE THE TEMPERAMENT TO WEAR BLACK?

You are about to embark on a chapter of self discovery. Understanding your true colors begins here, with your inherited personality traits. What better place to start than at the interesting Personality Questionnaire, which will ask you to write down answers about who you really are. Not what someone else wants you to be, or how you think you should reply. Spend some time thinking about your responses and how, maybe they differ now from how you might have answered in your past. Honesty is the best policy. Done properly this will provide you with a fascinating insight into your true nature, which will lead you onto your true colors!

WHAT PERSONALITY TYPE ARE YOU?

The Personality Questionnaire in this chapter is designed to help you identify your seasonal type. Each of the four main "temperaments" has important qualities. You were born with tendencies to certain characteristics as well as eye pattern and skin coloring.

This is a subjective look at your general behavior patterns and there are no right or wrong answers, only how you feel. For this reason it may be beneficial to ask someone who knows you really well to answer any question you find difficult.

When answered properly the questionnaire should give you accurate results. For any question that elicits is a "sometimes" response, simply place a half as an answer and add up the results at the end of the section.

A strong secondary score can affect your results. If you have a combination of scores then look at which one is the highest. A difficult period in your life may activate a suppressed element of your personality, as depression can bring out the melancholic as one withdraws from life in order to cope with current difficulties. Other factors can also influence your scores like religion and culture.

Older women lose their confidence and energy especially when widowed/divorced and often answer yes's to most of the phlegmatic questions because they have gone into themselves and lost their enthusiasm for life. This does not mean, that genetically they were born like that, but through circumstance they have moved away from who they really are.

If your personality is a combination of opposites e.g. phlegmatic/choleric or melancholic/sanguine it may be that you are having difficulty understanding your own feelings so this information might be very useful to you.

Generally with this system, we have found that there is an extremely strong link between health and the temperaments, which relates to your energy pattern. For instance the choleric and melancholic types show more emotional volatility, with the phlegmatic and sanguine finding it easier to control their emotions.

Warm outgoing temperaments will tend to have warm outgoing colors, and introverted temperaments have cooler quieter colors. Treat the questionnaire as an enjoyable look at your inherited temperament, as this will help you to understand how you feel about color which, in turn usually relates to your skin tone.

There is only one temperament, the Melancholic that truly suits black. Their introversion and lack of ease with people makes them create a barrier around themselves.

Find out for yourself whether black suits your personality!

PERSONALITY QUESTIONNAIRE

SET ONE

1. Do people tend to confide in you but rarely seem to listen to your problems?
2. Do you speak so softly you are often asked to repeat yourself?
3. Are you often tempted to be dishonest about your true feelings in order to avoid an argument?
4. In large groups of friends do you find yourself watching and listening rather than actively joining in?
5. Do you find it easy to be careful with money?
6. Do you dislike it when others try to involve you in their plans?
7. When people confide in you, do you find it hard to keep a secret?
8. Do you enjoy fiddly or detailed work which requires patience?
9. (Female) - Is it a bit of an effort for you to wear make-up on a daily basis
   (Male) - Is it a bit of an effort for you to spend time upon your appearance?
10. Do you find it difficult to muster the energy to get involved in a new project?

SET TWO

1. Generally speaking, do you prefer to be out and about rather than spending a great deal of time at home?
2. Do you find yourself doing a lot of talking in company?
3. Do you like to spread yourself around a number of friends rather than just one specific person?
4. Do you blush easily or have a tendency to red cheeks or

broken veins?

5. Do you feel that you are quite witty with things popping out of your mouth when you least expect it?
6. Is your general attitude to life optimistic?
7. Are you attracted to bright and exciting colors?
8. Do you tend to get carried away with enthusiasm and take on more things than you can finish?
9. Do people think you look younger than you really are?
10. Are you the type of person who enjoys the changing of the seasons?

SET THREE

1. Do you tend to speak your mind in most situations and straighten out wrong ideas?
2. Do you find other people irritating, especially when they disagree with your opinions?
3. When a friend suggests something new, is your first reaction often negative?
4. Are you often accused of being stubborn – even by people who are not close members of your family?
5. Do you frequently find yourself in charge of committees – or organizing other people in order to get things done?
6. Do you find you finish jobs quickly and need to move onto something else rapidly?
7. Do you find it difficult to give up on a project even if it is not going according to plan?
8. Is your energy level high, to the point that you can't really relax?
9. Do people often misunderstand you and feel you have offended them, when that has not been your intention?
10. Do you tend to get dramatic about situations?

SET FOUR

1. Have you often been told that people find you aloof and difficult to approach.
2. Do you have the feeling that people seem to look at you more than they do at others?
3. Do you worry a great deal about what other people think of you?
4. Do you resent the invasion of your privacy?
5. Do you prefer to wait for others to seek you out, rather than being the one to make the first approach?
6. Do you often catch yourself apologizing when you are not really at fault?
7. Do you usually check your hair and clothing before opening the door to a visitor?
8. Do you tend to opt for your own company at the slightest excuse?
9. Even if you feel sympathetic, do you resist getting involved in a situation where you will be depended upon?
10. Do you prefer work that does not involve you directly with other people?

Most "yes" answers in Set No. ......
Set One   ......   Set Two   ......
Set Three   ......   Set Four   ......

The Results - Your Personality Characteristics

If you had mostly "yes" answers in Set One then you have a Phlegmatic temperament, usually associated with the "Summer" season.

THE PHLEGMATIC TEMPERAMENT

A key factor with this good natured personality is a lack of inner energy and you may find yourself having to work harder than others to achieve the same amount of work. Especially as you find it very difficult to do a less than a perfect job, whatever you are doing. This is not really very efficient, as it often means that a small task becomes a large task taking much more time. For example the decision to tidy a cupboard ends up becoming a virtual spring clean. You may also be quite naturally slow moving, though precise.

Because you are driven by will power not energy, you can liken it to being a rowing boat. You get where you plan to go but it takes you longer. Because talking requires surprising amounts of energy, you tend to seem quiet and to talk quietly, causing people to ask you to repeat yourself. In group situations, you are often quite happy to be the observer, letting all the activity flow over you but observing and analyzing what is going on around you.

You can be very diplomatic and good at repairing other's relationships, by explaining people to each other, because you analyze people and situations. Your ability to listen well is greatly valued by friends, who often turn to you in times of trouble. You can enjoy 'pouring oil on troubled waters' and smoothing out problems between people.

You do not enjoy conflict and will avoid it if possible, even if this means telling a white lie. In fact you are not driven to tell everyone exactly what you think about things as your opposite temperament, the choleric, is. This is a characteristic, which saves much conflict.

Phlegmatics have great stickability. Having taken up a task, you can persevere with surprising patience until it is completed, not becoming bored as many others would. You will often enjoy hobbies which require a high level of manual skill and patience, playing an instrument for example. Craftspeople are often phlegmatic. When you want to start a new project, it frequently takes much longer than you planned, due to a combination of wanting to do things well and a lack of inner energy to drive you.

Providing you are doing work which suits you (jobs, which require care and accuracy rather than speed) you will be a valued employee and a good team member, not feeling the need to stand out from the crowd.

There is, an almost hidden, underlying inflexibility in this temperament, which can also be seen as stability. Last minute changes to plans can be hard to cope with and a conservative attitude to life comes naturally. You can find it difficult to say no to others plans when they are not in line with your own desires, then find that you have to do things you do not want because you did not make your feelings clear at the planning stage. Fortunately, you are usually a very good-natured person.

You can be careful with money, going to great lengths to avoid waste and finding it especially difficult to spend money on yourself, though usually being generous to those you love. This also flows over into the time you are prepared to spend on your appearance. For women it can be difficult to find the time to apply make-up daily and getting a man to go shopping for new clothes can be quite a challenge. Once people get to know you, your innate gentleness and sweetness of temper, makes you a very dearly loved friend. As you do not push yourself forward to attract attention.

Some positive personality traits: listens carefully, speaks quietly, gentleness, understanding, diplomatic, talented with hands, good imagination, easy going, dependable, practical, efficient and neat.

Some negative personality traits: slow to accept new ideas, makes friends slowly, slow worker, stubborn, gets lost in details.

If you had mostly "yes" answers in Set Two then you have a

Sanguine temperament, usually associated with the "Spring" season.

THE SANGUINE TEMPERAMENT

Your highest score is in the naturally outgoing and sociable, sanguine temperament. This indicates a flexible person who tends to enjoy life and people, and is optimistic that things will work out right in the end. Usually you pay great attention to those around you and although you enjoy this, it does mean you also need time to yourself, when you don't have to think about others, or their needs.

Your energy level can be quite variable, depending on how interested you are in what you are doing. For this reason you enjoy change and new challenges as the energy comes in to deal with them.

However, there are some sanguines, with a specific iris pattern, who have a very high level of energy. This causes them to behave in a similar manner to the more workaholic, choleric temperament, but to be less easily irritated.

The name sanguine comes from the Greek word for blood. Having 'high color' or blushing easily is normal, as it was this effect, observed by Hippocrates, which gave you the name. You may notice it when drinking alcohol or just being slightly self-conscious. Your skin may have a slightly translucent look to it. As the tiny blood vessels in the cheeks are prone to breaking, it's a good idea to dilute your alcohol, avoid very spicy foods and extremes of temperature. If this has not happened yet, it is a good idea to take precautions against it happening in the future.

This temperament usually has a strong constitution, with a tendency to make a speedier recovery from illness than most. Although you are not immune from ill health (especially as you are inclined to push yourself and ignore how you are feeling) your body does seem to be on your side.

This is also evident in the eye pattern. The classic 'Spring' eye is regarded by some Iridologists as the "pioneer's eye" and is associated with the people who get out there and make things happen. The strong constitution probably explains why sanguine people often look much younger than their years, and retain a youthful attitude into old age. Unfortunately, smokers or those who have been unlucky with their health or had a very troubled life may miss out on this blessing.

Along with looking young and having a youthful attitude, there is usually a natural curiosity and a desire to learn about the new. Taking courses to extend knowledge and qualifications are typical occupations.

It is not unusual for your many friendships to cover a wide variety of age groups as your empathy and lack of rigidity enables you to get on well with people who differ from yourself. However, some people do not approve of this youthful attitude to life and may call you childish. Childlike is a better word and describes the underlying light hearted, curious and joyful way in which you approach life when all is going well.

Your optimism and energy can cause you to take on more than you can manage in the time at your disposal. Learning to control this characteristic is very useful, in fact learning just to say no. Your communication skills and naturally outgoing temperament make you good in jobs, which require people skills e.g. teaching or selling. There is generally a love of color and often a better than usual ability to hold a color in your head for matching.

Some positive personality traits: curious, smiles often, friendly, good humor, witty, good conversationalist, optimistic, enthusiastic, empathy with others, kind, energetic.

Some negative personality traits: undecided, speaks without thinking, fails to plan ahead, takes on too many projects, manipulative, overly talkative.

If you had mostly "yes" answers in Set Three then you are

have a Choleric temperament, usually associated with the "Autumn" season.

THE CHOLERIC TEMPERAMENT

This powerful personality with a strongly outgoing tendency is often a high achiever. Partly this comes from a surfeit of energy, which causes others to accuse you of being a workaholic. Unlike many people, your energy level is always high and you do find it difficult to relax. Think of it like being a speedboat where the energy comes from the inner engine and is always there, driving you along.

You are usually well organized in your home and work life, and if circumstances bring you into committees you will usually end up taking charge in order to get things done. However, you can be impatient with others as you do not really understand why they are so different from you. This is because you are so busy getting on with things that you do not tend to spend time analyzing situations.

Often described as a "self starter" (much valued in business) you have much more confidence in your own ideas than those of others. This is why you tend to dismiss new ideas when others present them. You may find yourself re-examining your first reaction at a later date however.

You are very straightforward and people always know where they are with you. This may cause problems, as people do not always want to know what you think. However, you can be quite good at dealing with these problems, as you like to bring things out into the open and get things straight. You make a very good and loyal friend.

When you decide to do something, difficulties will bring out your stubborn side ensuring you stick at it, even if with hindsight, you might have been wise to give up sooner. This is an interesting characteristic, which means you may sometimes 'pull it off' against all odds. You hate injustice and this can be where the above characteristic is useful.

People in politics will always need to have some of this temperament in their make up, even if it is not their primary group. In fact as a secondary influence on the sanguine type, it can be very successful combination in public life.

Anyone with your amount of energy will always want to be on the move, making things happen. This can mean that you have quite a dramatic life style. Moving house or even country quite frequently. Possibly also changing relationships more often than is usual.

A disadvantage of having driving energy is that you find it really hard to relax and this is not a good thing. Health problems relating to wear and tear on the body are quite common but as you are so self motivated, only you can find a way to deal with this problem. This is recognized as a Type A personality. You rarely take your family's (or even your doctor's) advice, although in this case they usually know better than you do. Learning to meditate, possibly with the help of audiotapes, may be a possible solution. Even taking up a hobby which can be done sitting down.

Some positive personality traits: makes decisions fast, dependable, energetic, works hard, loyal, self disciplined, confident, plans ahead, organized, leads, gets job done.

Some negative personality traits: disagreeable, stubborn, easy irritated, hurts others feelings, takes over in group situations.

If you had mostly "yes" answers in Set Four then you are have a Melancholic temperament, usually associated with the "Winter" season.

THE MELANCHOLIC TEMPERAMENT

This is a complex temperament, which can make life seem very hard. You are a natural perfectionist and so are always striving to bring things up to your standard. You have strong feelings and can be very disappointed when others do not reach the same standard whether in work or friendship.

Because of past disappointments and a natural inclination, you do not make friends easily, preferring to wait for people to come to you and prove themselves. However, you can be a loyal and reliable friend once that has been achieved, and are even prepared to make sacrifices for them. It is this trait of waiting for others to make the first move, which can be seen as aloofness.

Without being aware of it you are putting up a barrier, which some will not attempt to cross as they do not appreciate the rewards of doing so. Having succeeded in becoming your friend, you will still tend to leave it to them to keep up the contact and prove their affection.

In company you may be quite self-conscious, feeling that people are looking at you and on a bad day that they are being critical. This is rarely the case, but it is how you feel. You very much want people to think well of you and this may be why you are usually impeccably presented. The female taking great care of her make-up and hair and both male and female dressing well.

You are inwardly aware that you are a truly special person, often with many talents, but you still tend towards low self-esteem and may need lots of encouragement. Unfortunately, because you are introverted, you do not really understand how outgoing people behave and you can be hurt by behavior, which may seem neglectful.

Melancholics, though analytical, rarely realize that they are setting these situations up due to their natural reserve. Actually all that is happening is that due to the busyness of everyday life, extroverts can fail to pay you the attention you feel you deserve. Try not to take these things too personally, and especially try not to dwell on the memory, as it is rarely intentional.

Works of art can often trigger your deepest feelings: paintings, music, theatre, poetry. You may be intensely artistic. You have the ability to concentrate and analyze, and as you need a lot of time alone, creativity may be a natural outlet. However, your perfectionist aspect means you set very high standards. This quest for perfection can severely limit any feelings of satisfaction as you often feel you could have done better.

Because you analyze situations in depth, there is a strong tendency to see the reasons why things will not work. Sadly, people who tend towards pessimism are often right. Please try not to let this stop you being a little more adventurous at times.

You have a strong leaning towards conservatism and may carry this over into your clothes, often taking the safe option.

Some positive personality traits: natural poise, loyal, good listener, truthful, sensitive, creative, perfectionist, analytical, faithful, dependable, self sacrificing, reserved.

Some negative personality traits: self centered, worries about what others think, lacks confidence, neglects friends, pessimistic, expects perfection from others.

CHAPTER SIX

DO YOU HAVE THE GENETIC COLOURING TO WEAR BLACK?

Now that you have discovered what personality type you are, let us look at the inherited genetics that will determine your true colors. This is a self help chapter that guides you step by step on how to do your own personal color analysis. By taking a detailed look into your eyes and then draping colors to reflect up onto your face, you will find out which skin tone you have. This will provide you with the information you have been looking for – what your true colors are and whether they include black?

THE EYES

It is fascinating to know that from the pattern of your eyes you will be able to learn what season you belong to and whether you have a cool or warm skin tone. Many of you will never have looked intensely into your eyes, you may believe you have a pure blue eyes for instance, and have been surprised when your eyes sometimes look green. The answer probably lies in the fact that when you do look closely at your eyes you will notice some yellow present. Hence giving you a "green" appearance, and indicating a Spring golden based complexion.

The pattern and colors of the eyes reveal not only your main season but often the influences of your secondary season if you have one. Finding out whether you have a warm or cool skin tone is key to understanding your colors and whether you can wear black well.

Here's how you are going to see inside your own eye to determine the pattern and real colors inside.

First, stand in front of a well-lit mirror or if possible (and preferable) get a small hand mirror and get as close to a window with natural sunlight coming through. If you still cannot see, then get a magnifying glass, or ask someone else to look into your eyes. Make sure you examine both your eyes as often the pattern will differ and may not be as clear as the other. Two eyes are never exactly the same but they will correspond to each others season.

Look closely at both your eyes and you will be able to see the following:

1. White around the iris
2. Colored iris
3. Black pupil

The most important part to look at in detail is the colored iris. You will see that your eyes are not one solid color so start by looking at what surrounds the pupil. This is where you will notice the pattern. For example a sunburst of color or some crypts, petal like shapes or maybe even some straight lines resembling the spokes on a wheel.

Look closely at the drawing of the structure of the iris and iris features. These illustrations will help you to determine what type of pattern(s) your eyes have.

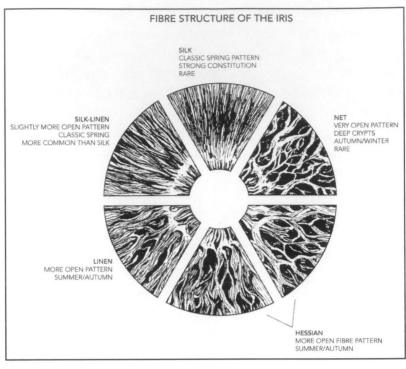

FIBRE STRUCTURE OF THE IRIS

SILK
CLASSIC SPRING PATTERN
STRONG CONSTITUTION
RARE

SILK-LINEN
SLIGHTLY MORE OPEN PATTERN
CLASSIC SPRING
MORE COMMON THAN SILK

NET
VERY OPEN PATTERN
DEEP CRYPTS
AUTUMN/WINTER
RARE

LINEN
MORE OPEN PATTERN
SUMMER/AUTUMN

HESSIAN
MORE OPEN FIBRE PATTERN
SUMMER/AUTUMN

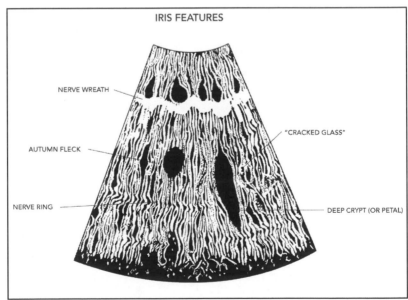

IRIS FEATURES

NERVE WREATH

AUTUMN FLECK

NERVE RING

"CRACKED GLASS"

DEEP CRYPT (OR PETAL)

BASIC EYE PATTERNS WHICH INDICATE HEALTH, TEMPERAMENT AND UNDERLYING SKIN TONE.

Without color photographs it is impossible to really introduce you to the amazing world of eye patterns, so our illustrator has produced drawings which will point you in the direction of basic differences. These will give you clues to look for, but you will need an Iridologist or a consultant using the Colourflair system to analyze accurately.

There are only two basic types of eye, though you would never guess this from the amazing variety of patterns and colors, when you start looking at the iris in detail. For people originating from cooler parts of the world, the usual eye has a blue iris with fibers, as in illustrations 1   4. However, many colors can cover the basic fibers, which then appear in a variety of shades from grey, green, gold and brown in a variety of mixes. The iris may also have a dark rim, not illustrated.

These patterns also relate to health and are how Iridologists deduce the needs of their clients. Because the iris changes with health, when the eye pattern does not relate to the temperament and skin tone, there are health problems to be dealt with.

The other eye pattern is the true brown, fibreless type. These relate to climate as the brown eye is protective from the ultra violet light of the sun. See illustrations 5 – 7. This type is also common in Chinese people and because we travel so much both patterns can turn up unexpectedly in different parts of the world.

BLUE EYES

Pattern one illustrates the sanguine eye, a pattern we frequently see, though some Iridologists think it no longer exists, as due to its indications of good health, people with this pattern rarely need to see an Iridologist.

This is a blue eye with quite a close nerve wreath around the pupil and close fibers stretching out to the rim, sometimes straight, sometimes slightly crooked, as we illustrate. There are many shades of blue, from very pale as in Scandinavian countries to quite deep, often with touches of gold spreading out into the fibers, causing a greenish tone. There can also be a haze of white over parts of the iris. See also 'silk' and 'silk linen' illustrated as Iris Structure.

Pattern two illustrates the pointers to look for with the phlegmatic (and sometimes choleric) eye. Fibers can be very higgledy-piggledy, with openings we call petals. Usually the fibers can still be seen through the petals. However, deep petals showing through to the black can be an indication of a melancholic temperament.

When this eye type is blue it can be difficult to know whether you have a phlegmatic or choleric person until a full analysis has been completed. See 'linen' illustration of Iris Structure.

Pattern three represents the blue base of the decidedly choleric eye and if we were using color, there could be many colors bursting out from the nerve wreath and lying over the base. There is also a tendency for brown flecks scattered among the blue, though these may appear on other blue eyes when there is a choleric secondary influence. If the overall color is brown, it can be difficult to distinguish from true brown eyes and you have to look carefully for the fibers showing through. See the hessian section illustrated of Iris Structure.

Pattern four represents one of the melancholic eye patterns, distinguished by the spokes passing through the nerve wreath towards the edge of the iris. The indication of melancholy is that the spokes start at the pupil. There can also be many openings without spokes. These may be deep petals showing through to the black beneath as mentioned above and possibly a red overlay.

It is difficult to illustrate the wonderful variety of patterns amongst the basic blue eyes without color. However, looking into your own eye and those of family and friends, as well as photographs in magazines will help you to understand what we are trying to show you.

TRUE BROWN EYES

These eyes do not have spokes but a smooth, velvet like area from the nerve wreath to the edge of the iris. This can appear to undulate slightly and can go from a golden brown through all the shades until almost black.

Pattern five is the frequently seen sanguine version of this pattern. The nerve wreath is close to the pupil with very slight openings.

Pattern six although similar to above, represents the choleric temperament. This has many deep breaks surrounding the pupil and the nerve wreath may extend slightly further away towards the iris rim.

Pattern seven these are the melancholic indications on basically similar eyes to those described above, but with dramatic spokes passing through the nerve wreath from the pupil towards the rim.

Although we occasionally find a person with a true brown eye with a tendency towards the phlegmatic temperament, we have not so far found that they can wear the cool pastel colors of the phlegmatic Summer range.

It is interesting that, despite the amazing depth of Chinese knowledge in medically related matters, they have never investigated Iridology. Presumably there is not enough information to be gathered from the true brown eye.

Pattern One

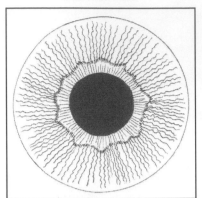

Pattern Four

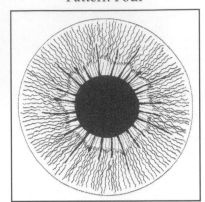

Pattern Two

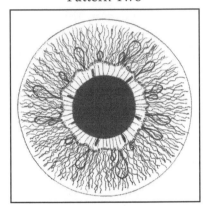

Pattern Five

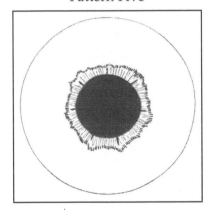

Pattern Three

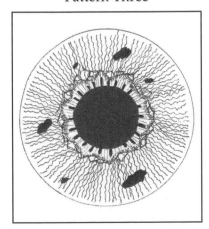

Pattern Six

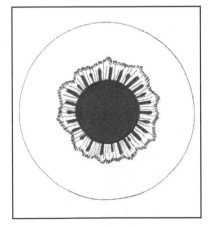

Pattern Seven

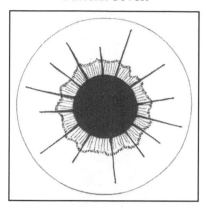

Summer Eye Pattern

The most distinctive Summer Pattern is the Cracked Glass effect. The white fibers will appear to be matted and interwoven and it is difficult to follow a fibre from nerve wreath to edge. The entire iris has the shattered look with little lines going everywhere. A good description of summer eyes might be the likeness of waves in water.

If you have Summer eyes then black is not within your color range.

Spring Eye Pattern

There are two main categories for a Spring eye color, and these are:

Basic Blue Eye Pattern:-
The classic spring pattern is straight and very neat looking like "well combed" hair fibers, which is known as a tight or close fibre pattern.

The other classic look of a blue Spring eye is the "golden sunburst" that looks like sunlight coming from a small space that surrounds the pupil. This pattern does not have to be connected all the way round. The golden overlay on a blue eye will give the impression of a blue-green coloring. Even tiny amounts of gold or yellow coloring are significant and indicate a yellow skin tone.

Basic Brown Eye Pattern:-
The pure Spring brown eye has a smooth, velvety appearance, free of significant patterns. Inside the nerve wreath the fibers will appear close together.

However, be careful. If there are deep openings in a brown eye, showing through to the black amongst the fibers and its is not clear patterned, this may well indicate an Autumn skin tone and not Spring.

If you have Spring eyes black is not within your color range.

Autumn Eye Pattern
The most useful indicator of an autumn eye is the deep open petals (or crypts) in a brown or green eye (sometimes blue). Usually this appears in a thick sunburst around the pupil or the nerve wreath and this pattern is called the "Aztec sunburst". It is like a many pointed star, with solid color coming directly from the black pupil, usually in gold, orange or dark brown.

If the eye is clear or opaque looking but has yellow, gold or brown specks appearing anywhere in the iris, then this may indicate an autumn influence but not the primary season.

If you have Autumn eyes black is not within your color range.

Winter Eye Pattern
Winter eyes have two distinctive patterns. Firstly the winter crypts, which look very dark because they are deep holes in the structure of the iris. However, the second and most significant pattern is best described as the spokes on a wheel. These appear round the pupil of the eye and a part (if not all) of the pattern will travel all the way to the edge. If it does not do this then you do not have a true winter eye pattern.

If you think you have a Winter eye, check carefully that your spoke(s) are straight, unbroken with sharp and not blurred edges – a half spoke does not indicate a Winter, and as this particular season is rare it may be that if you have signs of spokes then Winter could be a secondary influence in your eyes.

If you have Winter eyes, you can wear black in your seasonal colors, up against or away from your face.

THE COLOUR DRAPING

The Most Important Test – Can you wear black against your face!

You Will Need:-

A mirror large enough to see yourself from the waist up.

Lighting that is as bright and natural as possible. If you must be in artificial light then use fluorescent bulbs.

To be against a background that is plain and colorless.

To remove all make up. You need a clean face so get every bit off especially lip color and eye shadow.

To be clear of all jewelery round your neck.

To keep your glasses on if you wear them so you can see yourself clearly.

Black material (a piece of clothing or sheet big enough to put over your shoulders so that there is a large area of cloth under your chin).

Cream and white material (as above).

How to Color Drape for Black

Rest your eyes – don't strain them – ignore the material as much as possible and focus on your face.

Ignore your hair – if necessary pull it off your face with clips or a headband. You need to be free to look at your skin tone.

Position the black drape over your shoulders directly under

your chin, and make sure it is reflected up onto your face.

This drape will have a positive or negative effect on your complexion and this will be noticeable immediately.

What happens?
1. Does your skin look grey?
2. Has the blackness outlined and highlighted any unflattering feature on your face i.e. a large nose or jaw line?
3. Have your lines or wrinkles suddenly stood out?
4. Have you developed a "moustache" effect above your lip?
5. Do your eyes look dark and sunken?
6. Have your eyebrows become more noticeable?
7. Do your lips look very dark?
8. If you have highlighted hair do your roots stand out?

OR: -

1. Is there an absence of dark lines under the chin?
2. No shadows around the eyes?
3. Have the lines and wrinkles been lifted?
4. Does your skin look even?
5. Is there an enhancement of the under eye socket area and inner corner of the eye?
6. An absence of dark lines under the chin?
7. A clear and healthy complexion?

The Results
1-8   You cannot wear black well against your face – it ages you dramatically and is very damaging to your looks and particularly your complexion.

9-15   Yes yes yes – black is definitely for you! Wear it away from or up against your face, but remember to add other cool strong, winter colors to your palette too for a dramatic effect.

Color Draping for Warm or Cool Skins
It's Not Just Black.............

If you have just discovered that black damages your looks then you need to know that there are other colors with black in them that also need to be kept away from your face.

Navy blue is one such color. Many women as they age move into navy as they believe it to be kinder on the skin. Sadly this is not the case as navy has black in it. So does a lot of dark greens, dark browns and dark grays.

If you have any doubt about whether you can wear other colors well, do the self test in this chapter for black and you will see what effects the colors have on your skin. If they highlight the same negatives as black then simply adjust your wardrobe to wear them in the right way for your coloring.

The Effect of White on the Skin
When you drape white fabric under your chin, if you have a warm skin tone it will wash you out and make you look pasty particularly under the eyes and around the mouth area where the skin tone is usually uneven.

The white will make your skin look blotchy as it searches for cool white in your face. The face overall will appear lifeless and stark.

The Summer skin whilst falling into a cool season will also look unhealthy in white as it is too harsh for this seasons coloring; off white and cream are much kinder as they are to the warm Spring and Autumn skins.

On very dark skins instead of highlighting white patches on the skin it will throw an ashy or chalky color onto the whole complexion as if the skin has been dusted with powder.

White causes these effects on warm skin because the white

coloring thrown up on the face is out of harmony with the underlying skin tones. If you have the cool winter skin tone, white is an acceptable color against your face.

The Effect of Cream on the Skin

Once you have draped yourself in cream it will highlight to those of you with warm skins just how lifeless and stark white made you look. If you do have a warm skin then cream will automatically give your skin an even and warm glow. Your skin should instantly look healthy and golden.

Summers look particular pleasing in off white. Springs cream has a hint of yellow in it and Autumns have a coffee based cream.

If however, you have the cool Winter skin base then cream will simply make you look drawn and look sallow.

Other Color Drapes

Now that you have determined whether you can wear black against your face, and white or cream, why not have some fun with other colors in your wardrobe?

Here's how.......

What you are looking for are the changes to your skin tone, which will determine your season and what colors suit you.

Please take as little notice as possible of the drape itself and concentrate on your face, as you will see more. A color that is harmonious to your skin tone will also bring out the natural highlights in your eyes and hair, and you will be able to see the effects for yourself. Your hair and eye color will come perfectly into harmony when the right color is against your skin.

The best areas on which to concentrate whilst draping is around the eyes and mouth, as this is where the skin tone is generally uneven with patches of light or dark coloring.

The eye socket is really helpful as you can see the whole area to sink in with a poor color and darkness appear in the corner of the eye.

This effect is ageing and draws the eyes together, sometimes making a prominent nose seem to stick out further. These areas will be much less noticeable in the right colors as will blemishes, scars, facial lines, or unattractive features that you would like to draw attention away from.

What you want to see is an even, harmonious, natural tone to the complexion. The color should not make you look washed out, white and patchy, red and blotchy, or sallow, grey, old and tired. You are looking for a reduction in blemishes and lines if you have any and a lifting of wrinkles or dark areas under the chin or the eyes.

Reds

For warm skins, bright scarlet red will suit Springs, and the more orange, rust colored reds the Autumns.

Summers do not really like red as it can be too strong for their coloring and personality. A raspberry pink red will be better suited for this complexion.

Maroon and burgundy are Winters strong cool reds.

Wear red if you need some confidence and energy. It will always give you a well needed boost if you are feeling tired and it is a great color to wear on a date to create some romance. Physically red increases the hormone adrenalin in the body so wear it for any occasion that needs some action!

Yellows

Yellow is an unpopular color with many women, but in my experience once I show women with a warm skin tone how flattering it can be, they often change their minds.

Golden yellow can look fabulous on Spring complexions and will usually bring out golden highlights in the hair and particularly brown or hazel eyes.

The autumn mustard yellow is a devastating color on the

other seasons, but looks amazing on the golden, bronze skin tone of the Autumn woman.

Cool skins do not look their best in yellow because the skin base is blue-pink so it is not a natural harmonizing color. However, pastel yellow can look pretty on pale Summer skins and the acid yellow very striking on a cool Winter complexion.

Yellow is the color of the intellect and will help you with any form of study. It is also the color of self esteem and can lift your spirits as it is the perceived color of sunlight.

Greens

Bright lime green belongs to Springs, and pale mint to Summers. Olive and khaki green looks beautiful on Autumn skins and emerald is a brilliant shade of green that suits both Springs and Winters.

Beware dark bottle green. It is a shade with a hint of black and whilst it can be worn on dark haired women away from the face, it should be treated the same as black from an ageing perspective.

Green is the great physical balancer and if you are feeling under the weather it is a good pick up. It relates to the heart chakra so wear it to feel at peace and in harmony with the world.

Browns

Autumn women can wear most browns although chestnut is their best shade, whilst chocolate brown is a good substitute for black. Springs look good in camel and tan, and these provide basic neutrals for their bright pallet.

Summer has a soft rose beige, and Winters very dark brown, which has black added to it so all but Winter skins need to wear it away from the face.

Brown is an earthy grounding color, and looks wonderful with Springs bright red, Autumns orange and Winters turquoise. It can be kinder to the skin than black but should always be worn with a hint of color.

Pinks

Summer pink is softer than Winter's strong fuchsia. Whilst the summer tint will look good on a Winter being primary red mixed with white, the Winter shade is severe on a Summer.

For the same reason the softer Summer pink looks good on Spring complexions. It makes them look sweet and pretty rather than golden and glowing with health, fundamentally because Springs have a gold skin tone and not blue-pink.

Whilst peach is Springs best pink they tend to like Winters fuscia/magenta, which needs to be avoided if you have a high spring cheek color.

Autumn does not have a pink as their skin is bronze based. It is only the salmons and corals that veer towards orange that will bring out the best of this complexion.

Pink is the color of love and romance and should be worn in abundance when you need to be ultra feminine as it focuses on nurturing and is often seen as a sexy, girly color due to its association with flesh. To balance too much pink wear blue.

Blues

Blue is as flexible for cool skin tones as yellow is for warm. Whilst blues are flattering with blue eyes it is not necessarily attractive against the skin.

Navy is a harmonious color for Winters but warm skins take care as it has black in it and will have the same dramatic ageing effect close to the face. Summers and Autumns suit air force blue and Springs skin lights up in bright blues and turquoises.

Cool pastel blue suits Summers, electric and navy is for Winters, bright and clear for the Springs and teals for Autumns.

As a color, blue is physically calming and releases a hormone called oxytocin. It quietens the nervous system so is a great color to wear if you are feeling anxious. It is also the color of communication, so choose your shade for an important meeting or if making a speech – it will not only calm you down, but allow you to get across exactly what you are trying to say.

CHAPTER SEVEN

HOW TO WEAR BLACK IF ITS NOT IN YOUR COLOUR RANGE

If you have skipped straight to this chapter, then you obviously already knew that you could not wear black. However, if you have only just discovered from following the previous self help chapters that black does not suit you, then you will now know that you cannot wear it up against your face. If you do it highlights the signs of ageing and all the negatives that black shows up. The chances are you have found out that you have a warm skin tone, like the majority of women in the Western world.

Assuming you still want to wear black as most of you will, let me show you some different ways of continuing to do so, without affecting your looks detrimentally.

1. Do not wear black in a polo neck or crew neck - i.e. up against the face.

2. If you are going to wear a black top, wear it in a v or low-neckline. That way your natural skin tone will reflect up against the face.

3. Make sure you are wearing the right make up colors for your skin tone. This will go some way to helping you cope with wearing a color that doesn't bring out the best of your skin.

4. Wear scarves that ARE the colors that suit you. This can knock years off your face instantly and create the lift

against the skin to counterbalance all the negative effects of black.

5.   Wear colored jewelery, pearls or large amounts of statement gold (warm skins) or silver (cool skins) jewelery around your neck so that black isn't what reflects up.

6.   Put a colored stole, shawl, cape or pashmina round your shoulders if wearing that LBD.

7.   If wearing a black jacket then put on a shirt in a color that works against the skin so that the collar is what reflects up against your face and not the jacket. If white makes you look like you are in a hospital bed then go for cream - its much kinder on most skins.

8.   Black worn from the waist down can be flattering on waist, hips and legs provided you are in the best shape for your body and it can then be teamed with fashionable colored tops.

9.   Wear a boyfriend blazer in a color of your choice to instantly update an old black favourite.

10. If making a new LBD purchase try and choose a two-tone dress with color on the top or a patterned item that has black and other colors in it.

To see some examples of women wearing black really well without ageing themselves then go to
http:\\www.colourconsultancy.co.uk\book\photos.jpg

THE SCARF THING!

Many of you might be yawning at this point with the idea of wearing scarves. Color consultants have been banging on for years about scarves worn in lots of color shades up against the face, so this is nothing new you might be thinking.

Scarves do not have to be dull, plain, acrylic, scratchy, dowdy or old fashioned. The pashmina took the scarf thing into a fashionable arena where women had not been before. Beautiful cashmere and silks in stunning colors to wear in the evening to keep you warm without having to wear a heavy jacket or thrown casually over a leather jacket for added color and trend.

From there we went into major fashion labels – DVF, Missoni, Alexander Mcqueen, to name just a few. Stunning patterned designs, with leopard print, skulls, florals in wonderful colors; muted and bright. Suddenly the High Street caught on and there were scarves everywhere in all shapes – skinnies, long, neck scarves in wool, cashmere, cotton, silk but affordable, elegant and totally changing and inspiring women's wardrobes.

So, the scarf is no longer something resigned to Parisians, or the very elderly! It has become one of the biggest fashion statements and accessories that you can purchase. A scarf in your colors, that is the right shape and length to suit your bone structure and your height will last you a lifetime, i.e. will harmonize with your wardrobe and your coloring and allow you to wear your beloved black. What more could you ask from one small piece of cloth?

JEWELS, STONES AND METALS

Accessories have never been so big, literally. Costume jewelery adorns most high street and designer stores, so your choice of colored stones, glass and metals is endless. Lets be honest, black provides a great background for big statement jewelery – just make sure that you are wearing the right colors against your skin to counteract the negative effect that black has on you.

If you have a warm, yellow base then all of the golds will look fabulous when teamed with stones of amber, greens and reds. Pearls also look flattering against warm skins, particularly large ones, if they suit your bone structure.

COLLARS AND POLOS

What you wear up against your skin is key and any polo neck can be worn with black provided it's a good color for you. That way you get to keep the black jacket or coat but also combine a flattering color against your face.

The same is true of your shirts. The collars reflect light and color up against your face so its important with any black outerwear that your collars are in good shades for your skin tone. If you are at work or wanting a smart look that is not color based, then cream shirts with black are very smart and classic.

BLACK BOTTOMS

If you want to look slim and elongate your legs then wearing black trousers will do the job, provided you are wearing the correct style to suit your body shape. If you are looking for longer legs then wearing black shoes/boots will automatically give you more height. Black skirts should be worn with black tights and shoes for a lengthening effect.

Also, wearing a black belt with black bottoms will make your body look slimmer and longer legged which will look great provided you don't have a really short waist which may throw you out of proportion.

LITTLE BLACK DRESSES

Try and buy black dresses that are cut low and away from the face – even a small amount of our your skin reflecting against your face will make a difference. If you want to know how much, then take a piece of black cloth and put it up against your neck. Then slowly pull it down and see how far you need to go to take the black effect away.

Also, do consider buying dresses with colored patterns on a black background or a two tone dress with the color above the waist.

Wearing a block black dress or trousers and top worn low cut will look very slimming with a colored coat or long jacket/cardigan over it.

COLOURED TOPS

Obviously the key to wearing black but not against the face is to buy some colored tops. Cardigans, jumpers, blouses and t-shirts that can be worn under jackets and coats, or wear a colored jacket over black outfits. If you are not keen on color, choose off white, cream or one of your flattering neutral colors to go on top.

HATS

Remember that hats will reflect down onto your face, so if you choose a black hat be prepared for the black effect. Choose a brim with a color underneath.

MAKE UP

If you decide to continue wearing black against your face, then make sure your make up is in the right colored tones for your complexion and features. This will ensure that your cosmetics bring out the best of your features and harmonize with your skin tone thus going some way to negating the harsh, ageing affects of black.

Some Case Studies

Susie, Singer to the Stars

"I am part of a well known duo who are highly regarded backing vocalists. I have worked alongside The Who, Queen, Pavarotti, Lionel Ritchie and many of the greatest rock/pop artists of our time.

When performing backing vocals, I have often chosen to wear black. It was always a safe color and slimming. Nowadays, after working with Jules on many rock stages, I have realized that it's much softer on the face, to wear colors that go with my skin tones and flatter the face, giving me a softer look.

The heavy makeup is still great at times, but color is much more flattering than the blacks around the eyes. Dark colors can create darkness below the eyes, so its best to take the blacks away from the face...maybe wearing a lower cut top or dress.

As I get older, I find that bright colors give me a natural face lift and brighten up my eyes. So I may choose to wear a scarf around my neck or even jewelery that is chunky and bright. Taking the dark clothes away from the face, works!"

Michelle, Mother of Three

"Even though I have dark golden skin and black hair, I do have black in my wardrobe but I just try and not wear it near my face.
Jules showed me that black can make you feel slim but it can also age you if you wear it against your face, so now I wear colors and lots of them as long as they are the colors that suit me and keep black to a minimum. I also think that wearing colors brighten your day just by wearing them!!"

Fiona, Personal Assistant

"Like many women, I wore black as I thought it would make me look slimmer and more sophisticated. Then I met Jules - what a revelation. We spent about 2 hours together during which time she utterly convinced me otherwise.

Not being 21 I have some lines that show I have lived and these seemed to pop out at me when Jules held a black scarf under my chin.

Interestingly similar things happened when she did the same with a white scarf. It made me looked washed out, until she replaced it with cream, which completely softened my features.

What a difference, so I now know I am an official Autumn lady, with a huge choice of lovely warm colors, browns, oranges, reds, greens and certain blues, and many colors in between. A huge bonus is, shopping. Jules leaves you with a color fan that you can carry in your bag and you find you go straight to your colors, which saves masses of time.

I am completely converted and got rid of everything black and believe me there was quite a lot. In the words of Amy Whitehouse, I will never 'Go Back To Black'."

Charlotte, Working Mother

"With 2 small children and a demanding job (with a long daily commute), I just don't have time to plan my wardrobe and I need to be make myself look presentable quickly. I took advice from Jules on my colors and clothes because I kept wearing the same things and they tended to be based around black or other dark severe colors, which weren't at all flattering. Once I had seen how certain colors against my face made me look good even without the make up it was absolutely amazing, and I just couldn't believe that I had worn black for so many years!

Accessories were never my strong point, but as my budget was limited, and I didn't want to "start again", I put some scarves, jewelery and colored tops in my wardrobe, and suddenly my old dark suits and jackets took on a new life! I also learnt how to tailor the look if I needed to go out in the evening. It really transformed my wardrobe and was not expensive".

Elizabeth, Businesswoman

"I run my own company and its really important that my image is smart and tailored when I meet clients.

With pale skin, blue eyes and blonde hair, I never realised quite how draining black was until I started to show signs of ageing in my early 40's. When Jules showed me how hard black was against my skin and how much more make up I needed to wear in order to counteract the graying effect on my face I decided to change my make up to suit my skin tone.

This has made a huge difference to the way I look and so I started buying suits in grays and blues, which look so much better than black - softer and much kinder to my skin.

I have kept the black evening dresses that are cut low and not up against my face as I do like the classic look for smart events. However, I now get comments from female clients when I am in the colors that suit me, and this just encourages me to buy more of them. It is great to know that wearing the right colors can counteract the ageing effects on the face".

Karen, Interior Designer
"Up until a few years ago I was a slave to black. It was a staple that I couldn't do without, and truthfully it made shopping and packing for travel easy but it was BORING and too safe. Black is great and stylish for most occasions, and a necessity in my wardrobe, but I wear it very differently these days.

I NEVER wear it close to my face as it completely drains away my color and makes me look grey, older and sad.

When I wear black, I accessorize with color and I have expanded my wardrobe with beautiful blues, turquoise and emerald green being my favorites for scarves, jewelery, wraps, handbags, gloves and jackets. People often pay me compliments and say "That color looks so great on you as it brings out the color of your eyes". It is definitely not black they are referring too!"

Sue, Human Resources
I used to wear black quite a lot, particularly in my 20's and 30's and mainly for work. I have always had a black suit, smart trousers and of course the inevitable LBD. I wore black because it felt smart, slimming and easy.

After I had my colors done I was amazed at how much it aged me when I saw the difference in the mirror against all the colors I could wear. I suppose when you are young you can get away with more. Now I have reached 50 the skin tone is going and certainly the shadows and lines show. The black extenuated them to quite a shocking degree.

I am so delighted to have a color palette to work with now. There is something about wearing the right colors that makes me feel happy and optimistic whereas black and dark brown has a slightly dampening effect on me. I can honestly say it has transformed the way I buy clothes and accessories like handbags and scarves. I don't waste time searching through racks of clothes. I scan for my colors. If it's not me then off I go. Saves time and money. Also it surprised me to find that over time my wardrobe has started to co-ordinate itself, so I am using everything not shoving the mistakes to the back. Even a bit of black can stay if I wear it with the right color against my face, although I have to say I rarely bother, and certainly have not bought anything black since having my colors done".

Mel, Personal Fitness Instructor

Mel lived in black before she came to me for help. As she predominantly wore dark, drab shades she desperately needed a change in the way she felt and looked.

Mel said "I am one of those people who buys a lot of black because its easy to combine. This has to stop, or I will age before my time".

Mel turned out to be a Spring with a warm, golden based skin tone and lovely green eyes, suiting all the clear, bright blues and greens, purples and pinks.

She says "The change feels really uplifting to the point that even my husband takes notice of how fresh and colorful I look. Things can only get better!

If you would like to see pictures of Mel' s wardrobe before and after her color consultation then go to http:\\www.colourconsultancy.co.uk\book\mels-wardrobes.jpg

SO WHAT COLORS SHOULD YOU BE WEARING?

If you have done the self tests in the previous chapters you should know by now what personality type you are and whether you have a cool or warm skin tone. The following seasonal descriptions will tell you in detail what your true colors are for your wardrobe, at work and at home, including all your colored accessories and jewelery. It also covers what colored make up you should be wearing to match your skin tone. The colored fans will become an invaluable tool for you, as they demonstrate exactly what your harmonizing colors are.

THE SPRING WOMAN
Spring Coloring

The Spring complexion has a great deal of variety and can be anything from extremely pale to very dark. It may appear slightly translucent when pale, which particularly applies to red heads or Springs that are very freckled. You may have pink cheeks and a tendency to blush, and this may develop into broken veins when older. Do not be confused by high coloring from arterial veins close to the surface of the skin looking blue, this applies to the mouth and other veins. Many darker skinned Springs will have a deep golden brown complexion. The Spring glow has a vibrant golden quality which harmonizes with the warmth of your coloring.

If you have a sunny sanguine personality and clear patterned eyes then you are most likely to be a Spring. Your eyes are probably blue, blue-green, grey or grey-green, possibly with a yellow sunburst around the iris. Brown eyes exist with a clear pattern.

Hair may be any color. Redheads often have sandy colored hair, strawberry blondes are often Springs, along with very dark brown and black hair. When coloring your hair make sure you never use ash tones, only gold, warm highlights.

The difference between the Spring complexion and Autumn is that Springs often have a high color to their complexion - a rosy glow especially after exertion, and a skin tone that blushes easily. Most Spring skins tan easily and well to a golden color.

Some Springs have very fair skin and can be mistaken for Summer complexion. However, if you are confused try wearing cool shades against your skin and see if you look "hospital" bed washed out! A lot of women are "miss-typed" as Summers when they are really Springs and look a hundred times better in bright, clear colors.

When wearing your correct colors your skin will have a healthy glow and a youthful appearance, and a vibrant quality, which harmonizes with the warmth of your colors.

Spring Wardrobe

Your KEY COLOURS are joyful and outgoing, as you are. They are pure, rainbow colors, warmed by a touch of sunshine yellow. Think of new leaves and the early colors of spring flowers. They include most of the colors used in color therapy, as their vibrations are part of the light energy from the sun that we need to survive.

You have the three primaries: red, blue and yellow. These are then combined to create green, plus orange and purple which need some softening by white to make them work for you. The various mixes of red, orange and white give you the many blends of peach and coral which are very flattering, having a strong relationship to the mix of colors in your skin tone.

If you are dark skinned you will not be able to see this relationship so clearly, but the flattering effect will still be there. It is vital to be aware that having a darker tone does not mean you can only wear darker and cooler colors.

The brighter shades are very flattering to your sanguine complexion, however light or dark skinned, although this may come as quite a surprise. This group of colors improves more people's complexions than any other, possibly because they are the therapeutic colors of the rainbow. They lift off shadows and smooth the skin tone, helping you to look young and well.

In fact just a small amount of a bright color incorporated into a wardrobe can lift and enliven it. Do you have a garment in your wardrobe like this, which people have complimented you on, but you still don't wear very often?

Sanguines are usually strongly influenced by fashion and many of them have been 'hiding their light' in black (or navy) for many years. Also, when life is hard they tend to be drawn to the dark shades. Black is not the color of mourning in so many cultures by accident. Sometimes we have to mourn the loss of a relationship, health or even youth. At these times young women go towards black with older women choosing navy, losing their natural hopefulness and developing melancholic characteristics while they cope.

If this should be the case with you, then try a few small touches of your Key Colors with your darker shades and they will lift and heal your spirits over time. If they feel too bright to wear at these times, incorporate them into your surroundings. A beautiful poster, some pretty cushions or glass ornaments and just enjoy just looking at them. Also do not neglect to use the pastels of your colors as I believe there is a homeopathic affect when the bright pure color is diluted with white.

Color is so flexible. After all, we start with only the three primaries plus black and white and from these five colors come the myriads of shades available. This means that your family of colors (as mentioned above) which are primarily clear, warm and bright also includes pastel versions of your shades, as white can be added. However, black cannot be added because it makes them too dark. Dark colors, including black, can of course be worn but they should be kept away from the face.

The very important cream is your perfect neutral, and soft warm versions of brown like the ever-popular camel make excellent background colors to your brighter shades. In fact because the key colors are bright, just touches worn close to the face will make all the difference to your appearance. These colors are approachable, as you are too.

If your secondary influence is very strong, then look at the section in the personality chapter on that temperament. This will enable you to judge where your strongest influences lie. Which one is closest to your natural, from childhood, temperament, in other words.

We are all a mixture of the temperaments and people are a combination of the first and second influence as this mix is critical to how you face the world. A sanguine/choleric is very different from a sanguine/phlegmatic for example, due to the different energy levels influencing their behavior and response to life.

Spring Colors for Everyday
Bright greens, scarlet red, hot pink, coral, bright blue, bright yellow and gold, off white, cream, turquoise, bright orange, beige, stone. All tans look lovely teamed with cream, red, blue-green, peach, coral and yellow. Navy looks great with peach, red, bright green, blue-green, coral and yellow.

Spring Colors for Work
Off white or cream with small amounts of bright colors
Off white or cream with tan, camel, grey and navy blue
Navy blue, grey or stone with small amounts of bright colors

Spring Accessories
Shoes and handbags look best in tan, camel, grays and off

whites. Avoid black unless you are wearing a black dress with spring colors in it. Gold evening bags together with gold shoes look great for evening wear. Scarves should be bright and vibrant, and worn to suit your shape.

Spring Jewelery

The best jewelery for your yellow based skin tone is yellow gold. Your colored gems include turquoise, red and bright green and you can wear as much as you want provided you keep it light. Pearls also look lovely for a more classic look.

Spring Cosmetics

You probably have many discarded cosmetics in your cupboard as you love color and change and like to try out new colors. Your make up shades should enhance your natural vibrancy and balance your brighter colors. Yours is a "peaches and cream" complexion unless very dark.

Foundations

Your foundation needs to be warm and yellow/golden based either peach or beige in tone rather than rose or pink, and can be from the very palest to darkest of shades.

Blushers

Peach and apricot shades are most harmonious for your complexion but you may wish to use a more muted peach-beige if you are older or have very fair skin.

If you have one of the high colored spring complexions you will suit blushers that swing more towards the pink end of warm, but make sure you still keep the yellow base.

This will harmonize well with a cooler appearance of cheeks that may have broken veins showing through rather pale skin. Peach/orange shades are the best for blending in a high cheek color.

If you are a darker skinned spring lady then you will need a deeper version of these colors and red-brown or golden-brown blushers are best as long as the colors have vibrancy – this is most important.

Eyes

Greens have the right amount of yellow mixed with blue to harmonize with your complexion. They will create a natural effect on your skin tone, which may well surprise those of you who have not ventured into green eye areas before. Eyeliners in greens and neutral grays are best, try and avoid black unless you have very dark features. Browns are to be avoided as they may make your eyes look like they have conjunctivitis – not attractive!

Highlighters, whose aim is to reflect the eye in a flattering way should be in light shades of soft peach, cream or soft yellow/gold. Bright greens and blue-greens are also flattering and their vividness fun for parties.

Mascaras should be brown or green, but if you are a dark haired spring, use black.

Colors for Business

Browns and grays can be most effective in business situations but used lightly. Their natural dullness can be counteracted by brighter highlighters. Although the quiet dullness of these shades can be useful at work, be aware that they will make your eyes look smaller.

Purple eye shadows will look lovely because of the complimentary effect on your peach skin tone. Combine with gold for a great party look.

Lips

Peachy pink, coral and mango shades will bring out your best features. Choose a strength of shade that suits your particular coloring.

You can veer towards the more bronze-reds if you have darker skin.

The fans are shown on the back cover of the book but for a more detailed and clear look at your Colourflair Spring Fan go to http:\\www.colourconsultancy.co.uk\book\spring-fan.jpg

THE AUTUMN WOMAN
Autumn Coloring
Your complexion can vary from very light to very dark, but generally your coloring is rich. Your skin may appear to have a lovely metallic sheen to it and appear somehow thicker than average. You are able to wear a lot of make up without looking unnatural. Your golden/bronze skin tone probably tans well.

Like Springs your complexion has a gold undertone but your cheek color is not high colored but more gold or orange toned than the spring.

If you are a fair skinned autumn you may have the lighter colored blue, green, grey-green or any combination of blue and green eyes. If you are a dark autumn then your eyes may be brown or green with brown and gold flecks in them. Your eyes will generally have gold or brown coloring around the iris with an Aztec sunburst affect.

Your hair may be any color but is likely to have a bronze or metallic look to it. Auburn and dark blonde as well as very dark brown and sometimes black are also Autumn. When coloring, avoid ash and all cool tones, and keep to golden shades or copper.

As your choleric personality tends towards the dynamic and confident you wear your muted, earth tones really well and they enhance your strong personality.

Your earth tones combine so easily with each other and resemble the colors of autumn. You are the only one who can wear either light or dark moss green well which look beautiful with your browns and oranges.

Black is NOT in your color range, so learn to wear it well away from your face with your rich, warm autumn colors brining out the best of your glorious complexion.

Autumn Wardrobe

Your KEY COLOURS are warm and apart from orange are subtle and muted, redolent of the autumn time of the year. There is a stability in the numerous earth tones, from which your outgoing and sometimes impulsive nature could benefit. With many tones of brown as well as olive green, teal, air force blue and rich purple with some yellow in it, these can be quite sophisticated colors.

You share the various shades of peach and apricot with the sanguine temperament, together with the invaluable cream as a neutral. If you feel that the orange is too bright, then use either just small touches or the variations on peach.

You are the only group, which can wear mustard yellow, which is why you are called choleric as it relates to Hippocrates assumption that your "humor" related to yellow bile.

Your fan contains many of the colors, which are associated with creating a very homely atmosphere so you may already have them around you. If you are not drawn to wearing them because they seem, in the main, to be too dull then you may have a sanguine influence.

It can happen that those sanguine people who have a very high constant energy level can also score highly in the choleric section. They have a very different eye pattern and tend to find it easier to be patient with people than a true choleric.

Autumn Colors for Everyday

Orange, red-orange, olive greens, gold, turquoise, off white, browns, mustard, teal, cream and autumn colors in pastels combined with more vivid hues.

Browns with khaki and warm grey with red are lovely combinations.

Autumn Colors for Work

Browns with small amounts of brighter warmer colors, greens, gold, off white with any autumn color, touches of orange, teal, rust, navy blue with small amounts of orange or off white.

Autumn Accessories

All bags and shoes in brown tones will compliment your wardrobe. Black or white are not in your color range – wear chocolate brown or off white instead. Gold and bronze accessories are great for evening wear.

Wear scarves that compliment your warm, muted palette of colors, anything with an edge of drama or a sporty look. You suit tweeds, and paisley prints along with leopard and animal prints too.

Autumn Jewelery

Bronze, copper and antique gold compliment your skin tone. Silver can be used if your hair is grey. Your jewelery should have a bold, heavy chunkiness to it (unless you are very petite) with large stones in amber and dark green and big pearls or beads.

Autumn Cosmetics

With cosmetics a warm bronze effect can be achieved with a subtle metallic glow, which will work beautifully with your sophisticated look.

Foundations

Warm peach and beige shades in light and dark depending on the color of your skin.

Blushers

Red-brown and golden-brown shades will suit you best, even true brown will look great. If you have a very light autumn complexion then try a rich apricot shade instead.

Eyes

Browns and golds are really flattering for you but you also look fabulous in greens and deep blue-greens as well. If you like purple then the mauves are also within your color range. Remember the darker your skin the darker color cosmetic.

You can wear brown eyeliner round your eyes really well and are the only season to be able to do so. However, green is also an option in your khaki range. All variations of gold highlighter look good, as do light beige and peach. Only use cream on fair skin or it will be too light.

Brown mascara is best for your coloring, as well as greens and purples too. Black is possible but only if you have extremely dark features.

Lips

All shades of brown are great for you and bronze shades of lip gloss look fabulous. Orange shades are good as are deep warm reds too, especially if you have dark hair.

The fans are shown on the back cover of the book but for a more detailed and clear look at your Colourflair Autumn Fan go to
http:\\www.colourconsultancy.co.uk\book\autumn-fan.jpg

THE SUMMER WOMAN
Summer Coloring

If you are a Summer, then your complexion may be fairly colorless. You never have red cheeks or broken veins although a general pinkness can cover the whole of your face. You do not tend to tan well and should generally keep out of the sun.

When you wear the right colors you have a glow that has a soft luminous pearl quality, which harmonizes with your appearance. Your complexion will have a fresh, even tone to it when you have your cool pastel shades against your skin.

You do need colors that are light. Dark, deep tones will be too strong for your complexion.

Everything about you is delicate including your hair, which may be any color, from blonde to brunette. Although it is unusual for a Summer woman to have very dark hair, it can happen.

Your eye pattern is known as the cracked glass effect and is more often than not a clear blue and your phlegmatic personality is quiet and introverted, suited to your soft shades.

Even though you have a cool blue-pink skin tone, black is not a color that suits you as it is far too harsh and strong for your coloring.

Summer Wardrobe

Your KEY COLOURS show reserve. The rainbow colors are softened by the addition of white to many of the shades.

Think of cotton dresses hanging on the line in summer, gradually fading as the weeks go by and the sun bleaches them. This is where the association with Summer comes from.

Your temperament has a natural affinity with conservative blues and you also have the healing color magenta in your range. If your score in the Personality Questionnaire is very close to another temperament, the information on the secondary influence will be of benefit to you.

This will help you judge how close the analysis is to yourself. For example, this is a temperament, which many people (who are surrounded with strong and more determined characters or a religious belief that they should take second place in life) can drift into, to make life easier.

Also, women who have aged and gone grey (and sometimes also been widowed) may be drawn to these colors. It can indicate a loss of personal confidence, a feeling that you should take a back seat in life now.

These factors can influence your score in the Personality Questionnaire, causing the Key Colors to be out of harmony with your actual skin tone. This can also happen to naturally extrovert temperaments, like the sanguine or choleric, who have aged or suffered a loss of confidence.

If this is you then you will need to use the warmer pastels from your own colors to prevent your complexion taking on a grey tone. This way you can fade into the background while you need to, but you will benefit from the healing power of your own pastels and the great improvement they give to the appearance of the skin.

Summer Colors for Everyday

Off white, light blue, yellow, green, pink, lavender

Soft navy is a good basic combined with pink, blue, blue-green, silver-grey and lilac.

White backgrounds with pastel patterns and florals are very pretty.

Summer Colors for Work

Pale brown combined with off white or any of your colored pastels, navy blue or light blue, light grey.

Summer Accessories

Shoes and bags look good in browns that are not too warm i.e. yellow based. Keep away from black, but do use grey and blues. Navy blue is good for accessories.

Scarves in summer pastels shades will look very pretty up against your face, and small delicate soft patterns and florals will suit your feminine look.

Summer Jewelery

Pearls will look beautiful on you, particularly pink and you can wear them better than any other season, as they really suit your skin tone. You can also wear platinum, white or rose gold. Stones that are pastel and small and feminine are best, unless you are large in which case make sure your jewelery is in proportion with your size.

Summer Cosmetics

Your overall look is soft and delicate in coloring. You may however, have rather a lack of interest in make up and color in general, but I promise you it will make a lot of difference to your complexion and overall coloring if you get your harmonizing colors on your face as well as up against it.

Your cosmetics need to enhance and not overpower your coloring and keeping things simple is important.

Foundations

You need a cool, blue undertone which is rose rather than peach and you will probably only need light shades to match your skin tone.

Blushers

A soft rose shade suits all Summer skins.

Eyes

Lavender and muted blues and grays are lovely on your eyes. Pink and silver make lovely party make up.

The softer shades of grey and brown are best for mascara although black is acceptable if you have very dark hair. You may however, opt for navy or dark blue. Highlighters should be in soft pinks and creams and silver for evening.

Lips

Your most flattering lipsticks and glosses will be the cool muted pinks, with the raspberry shades being particularly pretty and will not overpower your coloring. Clear pinks are also good for the day and if you feel particularly adventurous bright cool pinks can be worn in the evening.

The fans are shown on the back cover of the book but fore a more detailed and clear look at your Colourflair Summer Fan go to
http:\\www.colourconsultancy.co.uk\book\summer-fan.jpg

CHAPTER EIGHT

HOW TO WEAR BLACK IF IT IS IN YOUR COLOUR RANGE

So, you have done all the self help tests in the book and YES you are one of the minority of ladies that can wear black well up against your face without highlighting any of the negative effects of ageing. You answered more yes's in the personality question-naire so you know that you have some or all of the melancholic character traits that suit wearing black and you have the cool, unusual winter coloring.

You can now discover what your true colors are, the ones that harmonize with black. Learn how to wear them to create the dramatic affect that suits your looks and personality. You will find out exactly what colored cosmetics will bring out the best of your features and how to use your accessories and jewelery to compliment your Winter wardrobe. Your fan of colors will provide you will all your cool shades and is an invaluable tool for your wardrobe and accessories.

THE WINTER WOMAN
Winter Coloring
You have a cool skin tone, with rose undertones. You may have either light or dark skin, but you do not have rosy cheeks. It is often the cool, confusing appearance of veins showing through their frequently translucent skin that may be the reason many systems classify Springs as Winters.

The assumption that pale faces and dark hair indicates a Winter is, in Colourflair's experience wrong more times that it is right. With a cool complexion it is unlikely you will tan well, but if you do your skin will tend to have a grayish look to it.

Your eyes are either grey, blue or combinations of grey and blue, or dark brown although usually not green. The patterns in your eyes have very dark crypts in them or straight spokes that follow through the entire eye from pupil to nerve wreath.

Your hair can be a variety of colors, including blonde but is most likely to be very dark brown or black. Luckily for you, grey and white hair is very flattering as you age.

Black is in fact your KEY COLOUR!

Unlike the other three seasons, there is the absence of dark lines under the chin, shadows round the eyes and any lines on the face when black is worn and reflected against your cool skin. The black added to your other Winter shades will harmonize with the cool blue-grey undertone of your complexion.

Winter Wardrobe

Your KEY COLOURS contain primary red, blue and yellow, together with pure green, often darkened by the addition of black. You also have the beautiful healing color of magenta.

When people are given this range of colors for fashion reasons, rather than because they truly relate to their personality, they often overdo the pinks. You are the only season who truly suits fuchsia, but you need to wear it in a quality fabric to look really good. A silk scarf or pashmina worn close to the face, as just one lovely touch of color, can work really well for you.

You also have pure white and black as colors and in your case these are considered "colors" and not just "neutrals". However, you are more limited in your color range than the other seasons, so it is important to understand that even though you can wear black, how to wear it to best effect.

A good rule for you is to limit your colors to two choices. Your unusual skin tone combined with hair coloring means that you do not need to distract from your looks with myriads of colors. Keep it simple and classic, as this look really does suit you best.

Icy colors look fabulous on you in pinks and blues, and dark green gives a real look of elegance. Royal blue can be equally stunning. Dark grey is a lovely cool color against your skin particularly when worn with silver jewelery for a dramatic effect. As your colors are cool and strong, you can add white to other dark colors, such as brown, grey or navy blue.

IMPORTANT POINT - PLEASE NOTE. If you have high color or broken veins in your cheeks, it is unlikely that the blue pinks will suit you. Because they emphasize the underlying blue of the veins, rather than blending it in, many people confuse this effect with having a blue based complexion.

In fact having high color is a very important aspect of the sanguine/Spring temperament. This may mean that you are not a true melancholic, but a sanguine who is finding it hard to cope with life at present. You may even be suffering from depression. If this is the case, you need the peachy shades (and not pink) of the sanguine colors to tone down the high color in your face.

Winter Colors for Everyday
White, black and white prints, fuchsia pink, acid yellow, electric blue, turquoise, maroon, plum, deep purple, strong red, and dark emerald green. Try not to mix more than two colors together at one time. If a warmer color appeals to you then wear it away from your face with black.

Winter Colors for Work
Black, dark grey, navy blue, dark green, white shirts.

Winter Accessories
Black, black, black!!! Shoes and bags can all be in black! Browns can be used as long as they are very dark and must match your clothing. White can be worn in the summer. Silver shoes and matching bags for the evening look stunning.

Scarves are striking in patterns that are geometric, striped and anything dramatic. Smooth and silk fabrics will appeal to you and colors that are strong and cool will look fabulous with your black clothing.

Winter Jewelery

Platinum, white gold and silver metal along with diamonds, emeralds, crystal and sapphire are all fabulous choices for you. Minimalism is your style, but these cool based metals look lovely with black and against your skin tone.

Winter Cosmetics

If you are a true winter with a melancholic personality you will be a real perfectionist about your image. Your coloring is most effectively enhanced by strong cool colors, which will harmonize with your skin tone looking natural rather than standing out against the skin in the glamorous artificial way they do on warm skins.

Foundations

You need foundations with a cool, blue undertone, whether you have light or dark skin.

Blushers

Strong blue/pinks will look the best and give you a healthy look, as your skin is usually colorless. You should be able to wear a lot of make up without being overpowered by it.

Eyes

All blues will flatter you and the stronger the better! Pinks and strong purples will also look good. It is the effect of these stronger colors blending in and looking natural that will confirm to you that do have a true winter coloring. Eyeliner can be black or grey and black mascara can be changed to grey as you age. Navy and blue make good party choices. Silvery highlighters in grey or pale pink are best.

Lips

Strong pinks and cool reds look stunning on you and will be really dramatic with your coloring. Keep away from the warm shades.

The fans are shown on the back cover of the book but for a more detailed and clear look at your Colourflair Winter Fan go to http:\\www.colourconsultancy.co.uk\book\winter-fan.jpg

CHAPTER NINE

MEN IN BLACK

This is a chapter written for the men in your life. Unless of course you are a man and bought this book for your partner and have managed to read thus far – in which case, you are impressive and your partner is a lucky lady! As the latter option is unlikely, we will go for the former assumption. That you are now a truly inspired woman, looking fabulous wearing her true colors and you want to share your new, acquired knowledge.

Women are not alone in having the right colors to make them look more attractive, men also have a seasonal palette. There is absolutely no reason why your man shouldn't look his best too! Most men are stuck in a color rut particularly because they have a more limited wardrobe due to work wardrobe etiquette.

For this reason you often find men in black.

Wearing black up against the face can be just as ageing for men as it is for women, in fact more so. Men do not have the ability to hide the dark lines and shadows with make up like women can. Therefore men are actually far more reliant upon color to make them look good, so getting the color right up against their face is in a way even more important for them.

BUSINESS COLOURS

In business, first impressions are most important because they are lasting impressions, and ninety percent of people will form an opinion within the first 10-40 seconds of meeting.

The most important rule in projecting a positive, professional image is to be well dressed. Anthony Trollope, the Victorian Novelist wrote "I regard that gentleman best dressed, whose dress no-one observes." For men wearing clothes not in harmony with their own coloring means the clothes will be projected – and not the men.

Looking and feeling good is confidence building. When men see themselves at their best, a sense of self worth will be achieved and this means that people around them will react in a positive way too.

The self tests in this book can be applied equally to men (with the exception of the make up question in the personality questionnaire). It may be that whilst you were filling out the tests for yourself that you recognized many traits in your partner. So now is the time to go back and do the same with them.

Having completed the personality test, they (you!) will know which temperament they fall into and these are the impressions they project to the outside world:

Summer/Phlegmatic Men

These men are likely to be kind, understanding, hard working and friendly. They will be an asset at work because they listen well. Co-workers trust them and they have no problems working behind the scenes. They are diplomatic, neat and efficient, albeit a little bit slow due to getting caught up in details.

Spring/Sanguine Men

Sociable and friendly, these personalities are creative, enthusiastic and make good communicators. They will love being around people and make many work friends, enjoying the sociable side of being in an office. However, there are times when less talking and more listening would be appropriate. They are a joy to have around with their good humor and general enthusiasm. Sometimes though it would benefit them to take things more seriously.

Autumn/Choleric Men

Organizers, who delegate well, these men are decision makers and can be true leaders. They will enjoy responsible positions but can be overly opinionated at times. Listening to others is important and delegating in a warm and friendly way will make them popular. An immense drive and determination can take them to the top of their professions.

Winter/Melancholic Men

Well presented and turned out these men are dependable real perfectionists and can sometimes be seen as reserved. They should try not to worry about what others think of them at work. Their natural creative flair and poise will make them friends if they allow their friendly nature to express itself. As perfectionists they like to get things right. They make good listeners.

MEN'S COLOURS – COOL OR WARM

If they (you) have completed the self help test in the chapter on genetic coloring then they should know whether they have a warm or cool skin tone. This is obviously key to understanding what colors they should be wearing to work and importantly whether they can wear black well. Their colors will also apply to casual/leisure wear.

For those men with warm skins i.e. Spring and Autumn seasons, they have a wider selection of colors from which to choose, some which may not be ideal for work and would be best kept for casual clothes.

For everyone, the brighter colors work well for ties. They are close to the face and therefore a great way to wear color and will lift and enliven the male complexion, giving a healthy and youthful look. However if there is a need to look older/authoritative then a dark tie should be worn, with a white shirt and dark suit.

Classic browns and greens are very "country" and have a poor research rating for business, unless of course they are indeed working in a country environment where classic tweeds would also be appropriate.

Casual wear should give vent to their personality and have no restrictions. However, black polo necks and shirts on warm skins will make them look older and washed out, so understanding what colors suit them is vital so they can be worn to maximum effect.

In business a high contrast between suit and shirt is always going to give the impression of more authority. Some colors (like black) can make them look very severe, whilst in others they will look much more approachable. When they know what these are then they can be used to their advantage.

Summer Colors

Summer man will have a cool skin tone, not likely to be blemished or have a high rosy cheek color to it. Their colors are conservative but should not be overpowering for this coloring and personality. Black is not a color in their range, it is far too dark for them so should be kept away from as much as possible, because it will be very severe and ageing against the face.

Suits – Trousers – Jackets

Light grey, navy blue, off white, denim blue, light brown.

Shirts

All pastel colors, off white (better than bright white), wine red, stone, white with small colored patterns, white with thin colored stripes.

Ties

Any of Summers pastel shades worn with an off white or darker colored shirt.

Bright pink/red, worn with off white shirt and blue suit.

Accessories
Shoes and belts in stone, or light brown, navy blue, grey, or off white.

Eye frames – Cufflinks – Jewelery
Silver or platinum metals, any soft pastel colored stones, silver or plastic frames in light pastel shades of grey and blue.

The fans are shown on the back cover of the book but for a more detailed and clear look at your Colourflair Summer Fan go to
http:\\www.colourconsultancy.co.uk\book\summer-fan.jpg

Spring Colors
Spring man's natural vibrancy comes through in their faces and their color palette is bright, warm and clear. They can however, tone down their colors for work but whilst the pastel warm shades can look great, they need to make sure they do not go into pastel shades of Summer. These can make the complexion look washed out and blotchy. Equally Winter's cool strong colors will age their faces and muted Autumn will make their skin look dull. Black is NOT within this color range but as many Springs love to wear it, they need to take note that their warm golden based colors should always be kept up against their faces.

Suits – Trousers – Jackets
Off white, camel, tan, navy blue, bright blue, light or dark grey, stone.

Shirts
Off white, white with spring pattern colors, print combinations,

springs pale pink, yellow and blue.

If black must be worn, then it should be combined with a colored pattern to counterbalance the effect against the skin.

Ties
Anything warm and bright in the Spring color range.

Accessories
Shoes and belts can be brown, camel, off white, black (if any item of clothing contains black), grey.

Eye frames – Cufflinks – Jewelery
Yellow gold, spring colored stones, gold or plastic frames in soft spring colors.

The fans are shown on the back cover of the book but for a more detailed and clear look at your Colourflair Spring Fan go to http:\\www.colourconsultancy.co.uk\book\spring-fan.jpg

Autumn Colors
With a more bronze based skin tone than the Spring complexion, these men do not have their rosy, high cheek color. They suit the earthy, muted tones of Autumn, and whilst pastels in their own warm tones can look lovely, they should steer clear of Summers pastels, as they will wash out the skin and take away the warmth. Winters cool tones will age their faces and this applies particularly to black, which is NOT within their color range. Whilst some of Springs warm tones cross over with some of the Autumn colors, generally their brightness will not look give them that coppery masculine look.

Suits – Trousers – Jackets
All browns, gold, air force blue, off white or cream, camel, dark grey.

Shirts

Off white or cream, camel, light shades of any autumn colors.
They need to be careful with pink it has a salmon or coral base.

Ties

Any Autumn colors: the reds, oranges, greens and teal blues.
Bold autumnal prints.
Prints, stripes or plaids in warm, muted shades.

Accessories

For shoes and belts, most shades of brown, tan or camel, navy
blue or dark grey.

Eye frames – Cufflinks – Jewelery

Copper, bronze or gold, earth toned stones; amber, red or
brown, green or brown eye frames look good.

**The fans are shown on the back cover of the book but for a
more detailed and clear look at your Colourflair Autumn Fan
go to http:\\www.colourconsultancy.co.uk\autumn-fan.jpg**

Winter Colors

So, these are the men who have the skin tone to wear black
against their faces without highlighting the signs of ageing or
throwing dark shadows or lines against their complexion.

They have the pure primary colors that are cool and strong.

My advice is to keep away from Summers cool colors as they
are too pastel for this complexion and the warm Autumn and
Spring tones will simply make them look blotchy and sallow, as
they are yellow/golden based and these men have blue-pink
skin tones.

With any of their clothing combinations, they should try not
to mix more than two colors at any one time – their striking
appearance needs to be complimented by wearing simple,

elegant clothes.

Suits – Trousers – Jackets
Black, navy blue, dark grey, dark brown.

Shirts
White, cool yellow or pink, blue or purple, any winter color mixed with black or white.

Ties
Black, white, stripes or prints, any strong winter colors of purple, red, fuchsia.

Accessories
Shoes and belts can be black or white, navy blue, dark grey, dark brown.

Eye frames – Cufflinks – Jewelery
Silver or white metal, diamonds or cool colored stones, plastic frames in cool grey or blue, silver or black.

The fans are shown on the back cover of the book but for a more detailed and clear look at your Colourflair Winter Fan go to http:\\\\www.colourconsultancy.co.uk\\book\\winter-fan.jpg

MEN IN BLACK - NO!!!
Men think that black is cool and classic but don't realize that as they get older black up against the face can be extremely damaging. Take a look at Robbie Williams; gorgeous as he is, wearing black is now ageing him terribly, highlighting all the dark rings under his eyes and the shadows around his mouth, making him look tired and drawn. He would look years younger if he started wearing some colors that suit his skin tone.

This is what Ian a Company Director says about his "black"

wardrobe: "I choose to wear black in both my business and personal lives....for different reasons...

For business, lightweight black suits work well for me crossing comfortably, and appropriately, between media and city environments. Usually I wear blue or white shirts as this combination with black allows flexibility to wear a tie or not.

Black suits are neutral but never unfashionable. I'm 6'2" and tend to wear slim cuts and black sets off that tailoring well. Socially I wear black shirts in the evening, (and black sweaters in winter). This works well with jeans or trousers.

I prefer black (or dark blue) for three reasons. First, I'm not a big fan of pastels/chinos for casual wear other than when near a beach or pool. Second, black, for me, has a hint of dinner-wear ....even when worn casually. And third, it's a fashion choice that I feel comfortable with. It is not for everyone (which is good), and the designers I like use black with clever detailing and cuts rather than using color to set them apart".

This is what Ian's wife says about him wearing black:

"Ian loves black. I think he has great style, and is always fashionably well dressed. Over the last few years and entering into his 50's, I started noticing how much better and younger he looked when he wore blue shirts and jumpers against his face. Black has started to make him look tired so I am now encouraging him to wear more color".

So for the men in your life who wear black, how can they continue to wear it without ageing themselves dramatically? Here are my top tips:-

1. Wear dark grey or blue suits instead of black.
2. Do wear bright colored ties, which will reflect up against the face.
3. Do wear white, cream or light colored shirts with black

suits.

4. Do wear black shirts with colored pattern in them.
5. Do wear black trousers with a colored shirt next to the face.
6. Scarves in the winter should be colored or in neutral shades with black coats or jackets.
7. Avoid round/crew neck t-shirts in black.
8. Avoid black polo necks.
9. Don't wear dark colored shirts with black.
10. Solid black is very severe, opt for stripes, subtle plaids, herringbone or hounds tooth.

CHAPTER TEN

BLACK BRIEF

Hopefully this book has introduced you to your true colors, the ones that complement your personality and physical appearance.

You will now know whether you have the introverted personality and cool skin tone to wear black really well into old age. You can feel elegant, stylish and chic wearing all the strong, cool colors that incorporate black in your wardrobe and also feel confident that these are supporting all the characteristics that make you feel truly good in black.

If you have discovered that black is not a flattering color for you, then hopefully you have learnt how to continue to wear it without highlighting the negative and ageing effects on your face, whilst still allowing you to get the physical benefits of looking good in it.

Maybe you have realised that your basic nature is not being allowed to thrive by wearing black and now your genetic colors can help bring you back into the person you were born to be.

Everyone deserves to look fabulous and feel confident about who they are, so the earlier you can start to wear your true colors the better. If you can share this book with someone young, just think of the wonderful knowledge you are passing on so that they may choose to look and feel their best from an early age.

If you encounter women or men that are starting to age, what better gift than helping them to understand their colors and how to counteract the ageing process by wearing the right shades against their skin.

We all need light and dark in our lives, as much as we need night and day. If we can truly understand how to use color to our best advantage, helping us through all the things that life throws at us, then we will be facing a better future, where we can live in harmony with ourselves.

Black has many sides to its nature – harness whichever appeals to you. Whether it genuinely suits your personality and coloring or not, understanding how to use this powerful color in your life and your wardrobe is key.

Balance black with the right colors and enjoy looking slim and sexy for the rest of your life without ageing your face!

REFERENCES

Author

Jules Standish
Colour and Style Consultant
Teacher – trainer of the Colourflair system

For personal consultations, presenting, talks on colour, corporate events. www.colourconsultancy.co.uk
email jules@colourconsultancy.co.uk

Foreword

Janey Lee Grace broadcaster and author of:-
Look Great Naturally - Without Ditching the Lipstick by Hay House
Imperfectly Natural Woman by Crown House
Imperfectly Natural Home by Orion
Imperfectly Natural Baby and Toddler by Realvision publishing
www.janeyleegrace.com
www.janeysnaturalstore.com

Chapter One

For details on *Pat Scott Vincent* and the *Colourflair* System, consultants and training www.colourflair.com
Theresa Sundt Colour Therapist, artist and author of The Art of Colour Therapy www.color-discovery.com
Diana Moran The Green Goddess www.primetimelife.tv
Recent book: Live Longer, Look Younger, Feel Great by Hamlyn
DVD: Easy Fit exercise by Stannah
Davina MacKail, Practising Shaman, Energy Coach and Healthy Living Expert. Author of The Dream Whisperer by Hay House.
www.askdavina.com or Tel: 020 8995 5003

Chapter Two
Gisele Mir cosmetic scientist – www.mirskincare.com

Chapter Three
Harry Oldfield – scientist, biologist and author
www.electrocrystal.com for information on Electro Crystal Therapy, PIP and Oldfield Systems.
Alla Svirinskaya – healer and author of Energy Secrets
www.allasvirinskaya.com
Alison Standish Colour Therapist
www.clearviewwellbeing.co.uk

Chapter Four
Dr Victoria Galbraith of Galbraith Consultancy, a chartered counselling psychologist, life coach and senior lecturer www.galbraithconsultancy.com
Philippa Merivale author of The Wisdom of Oz and Rescued by Angels and founder of Metatronic Healing www.metatronic-life.com
Faber Birren's book Color Psychology And Color Therapy: A Factual Study of Color on Human Life

Chapter Six
Sarah Jane Burrowes – illustrator contactable through Colourflair website
www.colourflair.com

Website, graphic design and photography by Ansell & Clarke. www.ansellandclarke.co.uk

Front Cover image of coloured lady by artist Vincent Poole. www.vincentpoole.co.uk

Recommended Reading

Janey Lee Grace – Look Great Naturally

Davina Mackail – The Dream Whisperer

Diana Moran - Live Longer, Look Younger, Feel Great

Alla Svirinskaya – Energy Secrets

Theresa Sundt – The Art of Colour Therapy

Philippa Merivale – Colour Power

Dorothy Hall – Iridology

Bernice Kentner – Color Me A Season

Angela Wright – Colour Psychology

Vivian Diller – Face It – What women really feel as their looks change

Howard & Dorothy Sun – Colour Your Life

Cynthia Sue Larson – Aura Advantage

Black in Fashion: Mourning to Night - NGV

Marianne Williamson – A Woman's Worth

Vicci Bentley – The Anti – ageing Plan

Harry Oldfield & Roger Coghill – The Dark Side of the Brain

Faber Birren – Color Psychology And Color Therapy

Florence Littauer – Personality Plus

BACK COVER ILLUSTRATIONS OF FANS IN COLOUR

SPRING FAN
AUTUMN FAN
SUMMER FAN
WINTER FAN

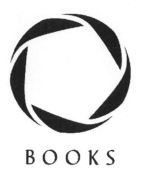

BOOKS

O is a symbol of the world, of oneness and unity. In different cultures it also means the "eye," symbolizing knowledge and insight. We aim to publish books that are accessible, constructive and that challenge accepted opinion, both that of academia and the "moral majority."

Our books are available in all good English language bookstores worldwide. If you don't see the book on the shelves ask the bookstore to order it for you, quoting the ISBN number and title. Alternatively you can order online (all major online retail sites carry our titles) or contact the distributor in the relevant country, listed on the copyright page.

See our website **www.o-books.net** for a full list of over 500 titles, growing by 100 a year.

And tune in to myspiritradio.com for our book review radio show, hosted by June-Elleni Laine, where you can listen to the authors discussing their books.

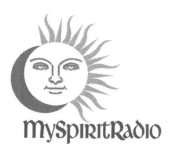